Excellence in Nursing Math Review

Tanga C. Elam

Copyright ©2025 Tanga C. Elam, BSN, RN, MSA, BAA

All rights reserved.

No part of this book may be reproduced or distributed in any form or by any means, electronic or mechanical, including photocopying, recording, or by any information storage and retrieval system, without the prior written consent of the publisher.

RN Math Excellence is not affiliated with or endorsed by any testing organization and does not own or claim ownership of any trademarks and does not claim endorsement by any third party. This published practice workbook is for general information only and designed to provide accurate and educational information regarding the subject matter covered.

ISBN: 979-8-9909316-9-5

Library of Congress Control Number: 2025908758

Printed in the United States of America

Sha Toya Roshea is my beautiful butterfly, who I am immensely proud of because you listened. I will give you my last breath if you need me to. Whereas I know that Jesus has you.

Claudine Perkins Ross always said, "Baby doll, land on your feet." Auntie Annie says, "And I love you more."

Jesus is on my main line, and I call him anytime. Thank you for guiding me and helping me to believe in myself. As I continue to find myself, and stay in my lane, I realize that I am enough for me.

Contents

Preface……………………………………………………………………………………7
Introduction……………………………………………………………………………….8
Role of the Professional Achievers…………………………………………………… 9
Traditional to International Times……………………………………………………….12
Administration IV Fluids and Drugs……………………………………………………..20
Pediatric Dosages……………………………………………………………………...32
Metric Units……………………………………………………………………………...47
Household Measurements…………………………………………………………........50
Cardiac Information……………………………………………………………………..66
Guideline of IV Calculations……………………………………………………………75
Section 1 Mcg / Kg / Min……………………………………………………………….79
Section 2 Mcg / Min……………………………………………………………………..101
Section 3 Mg / Min……………………………………………………………… 109
Section 4 Mg / Hr………………………………………………………………………..119
Bonus Problems………………………………………………………………………...132
Management of Diabetes………………………………………………………………...144
ABG Interpretations……………………………………………………………………..159
References ……………………………………………………………………………...168
About the Author………………………………………………………………………...171

Preface

Our mission of RN Math Excellence is to educate, inspire, display confidence, enhance critical thinking skills, and support a diverse community of students and professional achievers.

Dr. David Mayer, vice president of quality and safety at Maryland-based MedStar Health, said, "way too many people are being harmed by unintentional medical error, and it needs to be corrected."

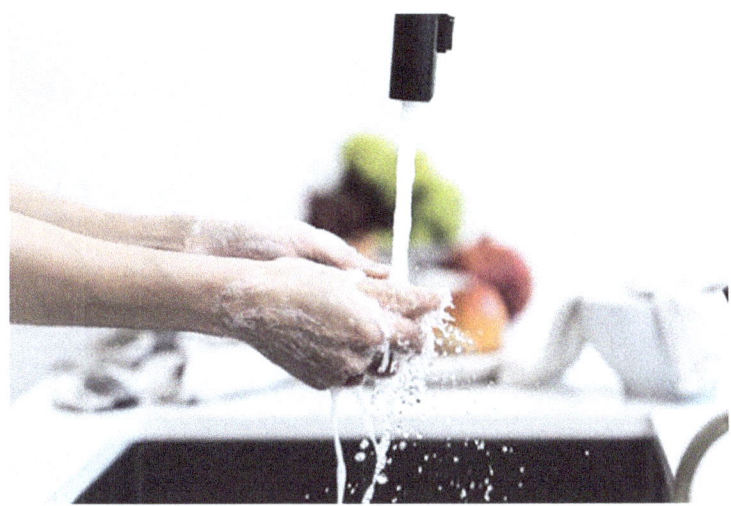

Introduction

This dynamic workbook initiates proven accurate adult intravenous (IV) math calculations by using the x factor with dimensional analysis formulas.

The best advantage of using dimensional analysis is the fact that all necessary steps can be taken using one equation.

The calculations of the x factor (unknown variable) are user friendly, completely individualized, and knowledge-based math.

Please use a calculation method that is most comfortable to you.

Whatever method you decide to memorize and use, the correct answer will prevent medication errors. IV math calculations can be used in most patient care areas of primary nursing, and one of the most extremely critical aspects of nursing is medication administration. Proficiency and accuracy can be the difference between life and death.

All brand and generic medications included in this math workbook are only examples.

Self-practice of the workbook will prevent medication errors which can lead to achieve personal and professional excellence.

This workbook is equivalent in relation to the Next Generation NCLEX ® (NGN) review and math courses specific to nursing and pharmacology.

Role of the Professional Achievers

Administration considerations are by use of infusion pumps, and the goal is to determine the correct rate to set the IV pump.

- Knowledge of types of IV sets and its drop factors.
- Regulating IV controllers, i.e., manual or machine.
- Mixing drugs and diluting IV solutions.
- Calculation of IV flow rates.

The student should be familiar with conversion units of measurement within metric, apothecary, and household system, including medical terminology and approved standard abbreviations.

- Review prior potential and actual adverse events.
- Educate yourself on new drugs, methods, and high alert meds.
- Clinicians who administer drugs to patients are legally responsible for recognizing incorrect and unsafe dosages.
- Check documented physician's order.
- Check medication ordered with at least two identifiers (for example, name, medical record number, and birth date).
- Identify the 5 + 2 patient rights: patient, medication, dose, route, time, right to refuse, and proper documentation.
- Calculations for dosage and flow rates *must* be double-checked to minimize errors.

100% accuracy

Do not use abbreviations.

Follow pharmacy guidelines and hospital policies to help prevent errors.

- Med mistakes often are from similarity in drug names.
- Confusion with look-alike / sound-alike meds.
- Poorly handwritten physician orders and communication.

The Institute for Safe Medication Practices (ISMP) has a list of abbreviations, symbols, and acronyms that should not be used.

It is safe to write out standard abbreviations otherwise it can become confusing and misunderstood and create medical errors. Listed below are JCAHO standards and suggestions of a list of do-not-use abbreviations.

CC	cubic centimeter or milliliter, 00
DC or D / C	Discontinue or discharge
HS	Half strength or at bedtime
IU	International Unit
IV	Intravenous or international unit
$MgSO_4$	Magnesium Sulfate
MS	Morphine Sulfate
MSO_4	Morphine Sulfate
OD	Once daily or right eye
OS	Left eye
QOD	Every Other Day or daily
SQ or SC	Subcutaneous
TIW	Twice a week or three times a week
tPA	tissue plasminogen activator
U or IU	Unit, zero, or 10
Ug or g	Microgram or mg

Statistics

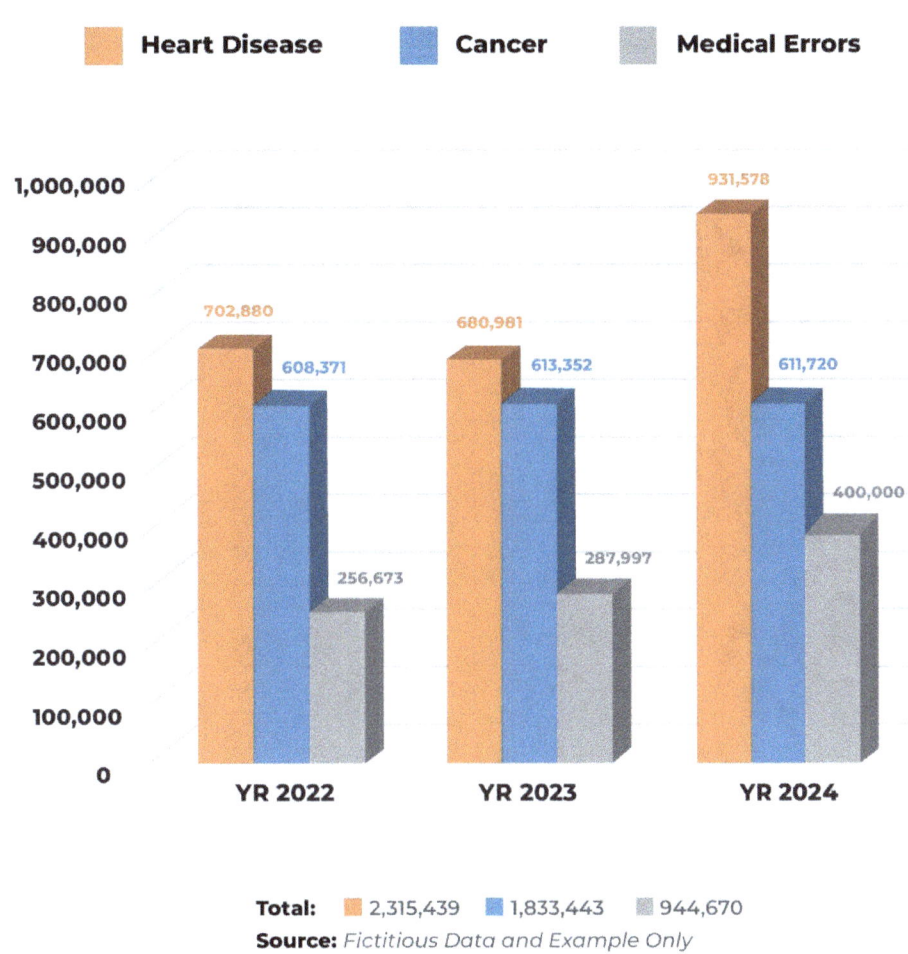

It is necessary to follow hospital policy and pharmacy department protocols to establish uniformity in the preparation and therapeutic use of potent drugs, which will ensure patient safety.

Medical error according to the Institute of Medicine is "the failure to complete a planned action as intended."

- Error of omission—failure of healthcare provider to deliver the best treatment to a patient.

- Error of commission—failure that occurs because of a mistake.

What is *sentinel event*? Any unexpected occurrence that results in death or serious physical, psychological injury, or risk of any of these outcomes.

TANGA C. ELAM, BSN, RN, MSA, BAA

What time is it?

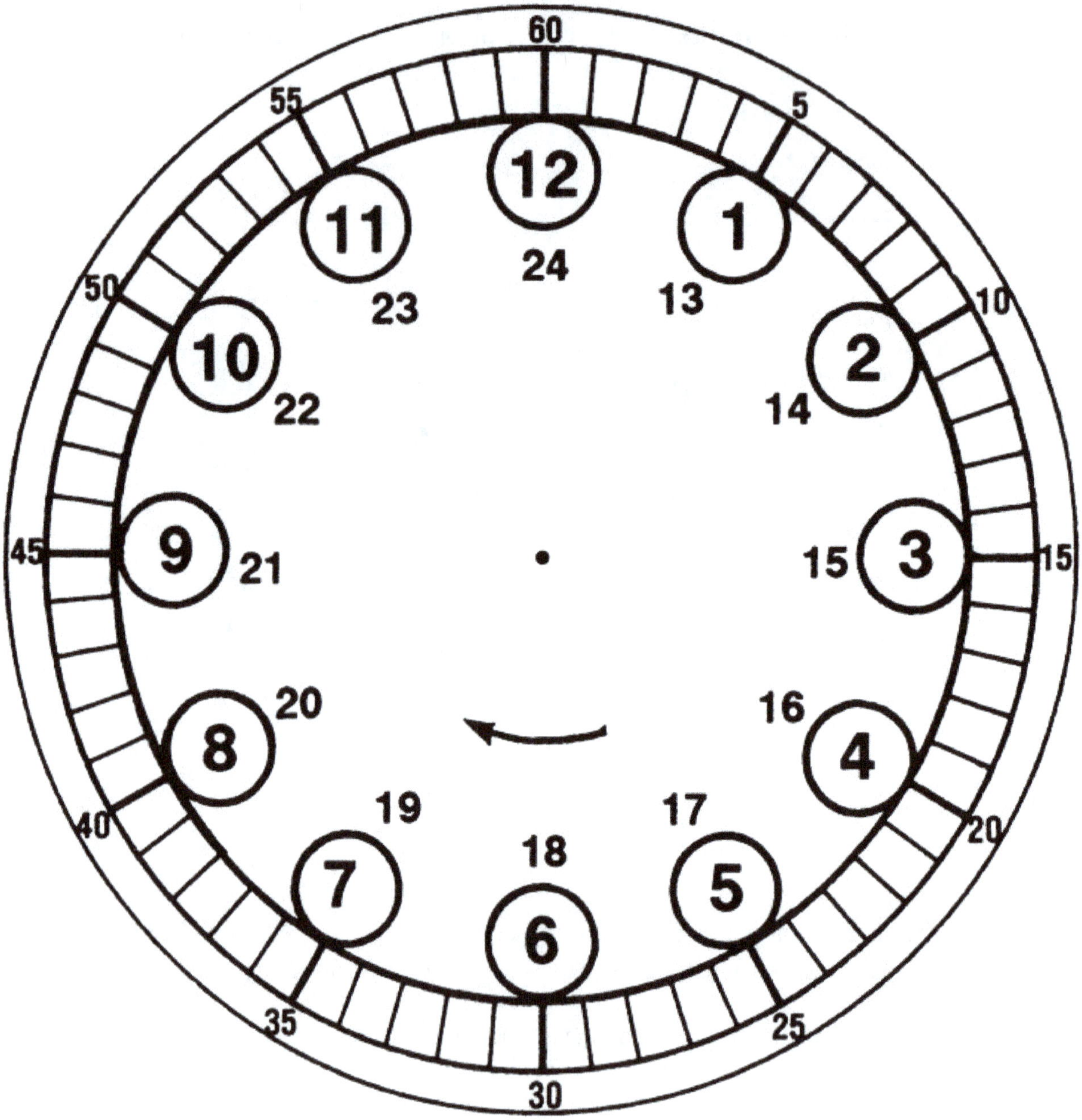

International / Standard 24 hour Clock
(Example Only)

EXCELLENCE in NURSING MATH REVIEW

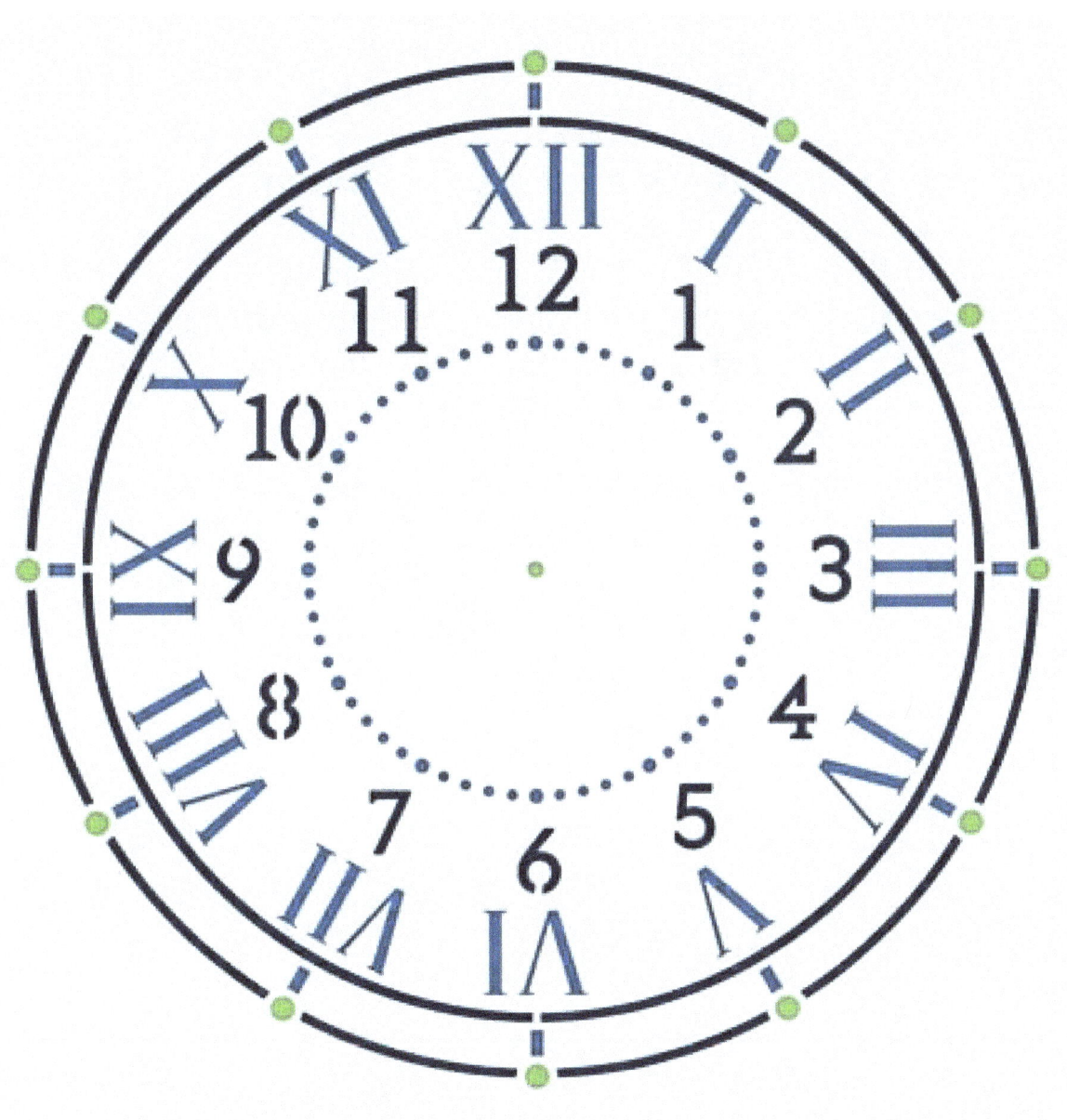

Roman Numeral Clock
(Example Only)

Roman Numerals

I	one	XX	twenty
II	two	XXX	thirty
III	three	XL	forty
IV	four	L	fifty
V	five	LX	sixty
VI	six	LXX	seventy
VII	seven	LXXX	eighty
VIII	eight	XC	ninety
IX	nine	C	hundred
X	ten	M	thousand

EXCELLENCE in NURSING MATH REVIEW

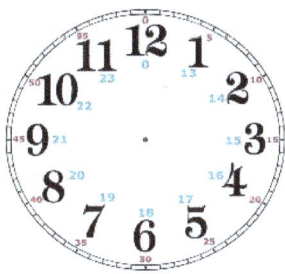

Example Only

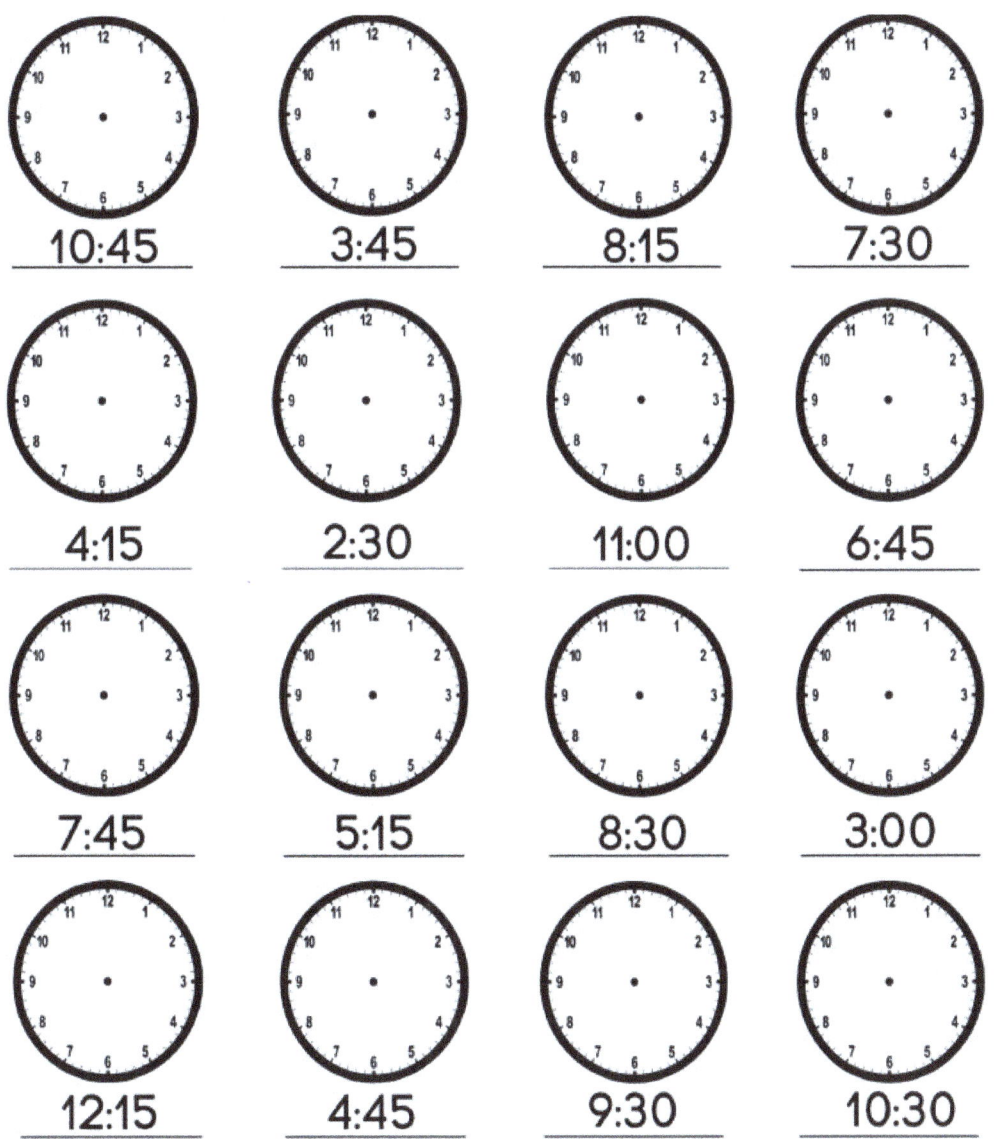

Practice labeling the hours and minutes for each clock.

TANGA C. ELAM, BSN, RN, MSA, BAA

What time is it?

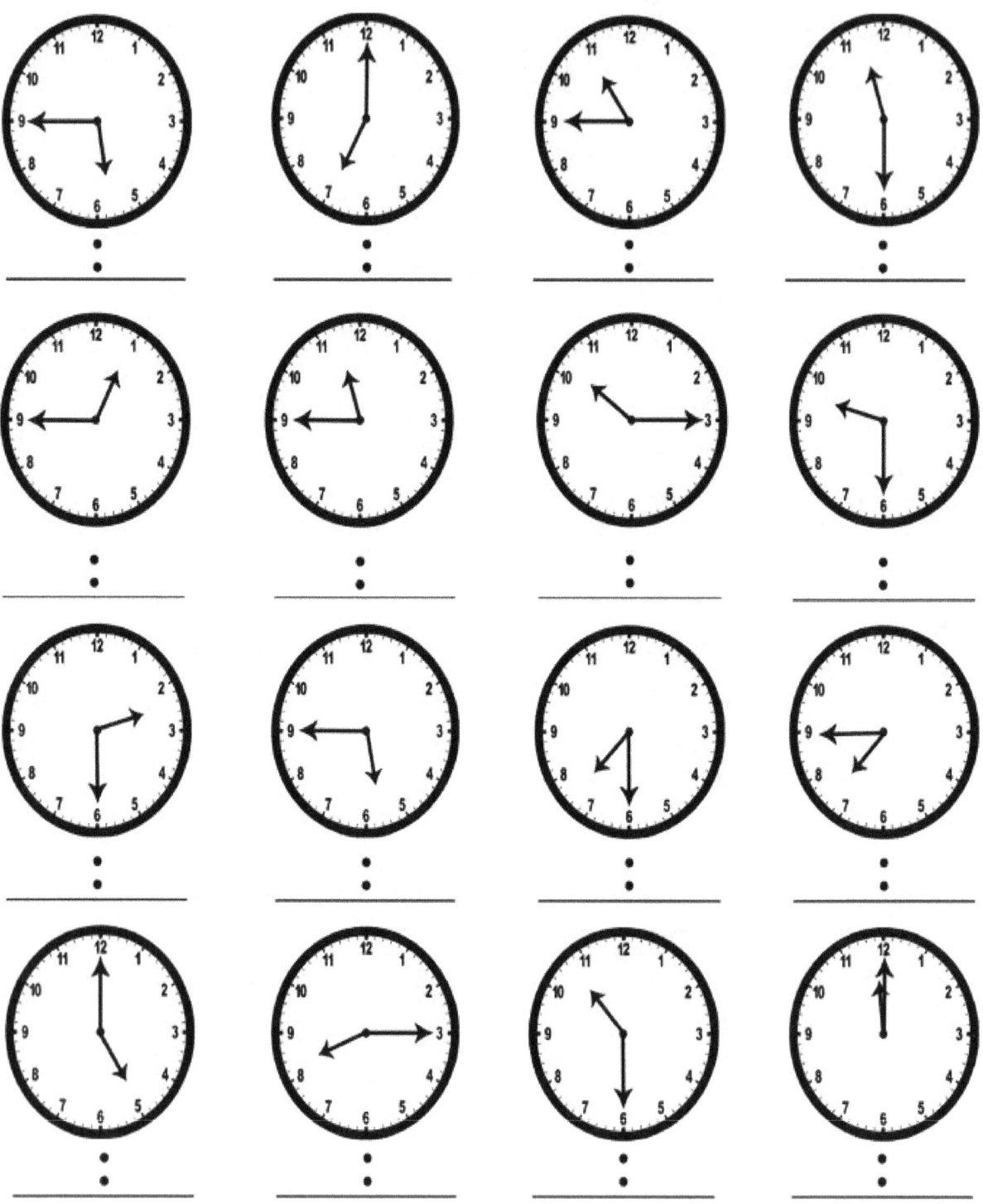

Example Only

EXCELLENCE in NURSING MATH REVIEW

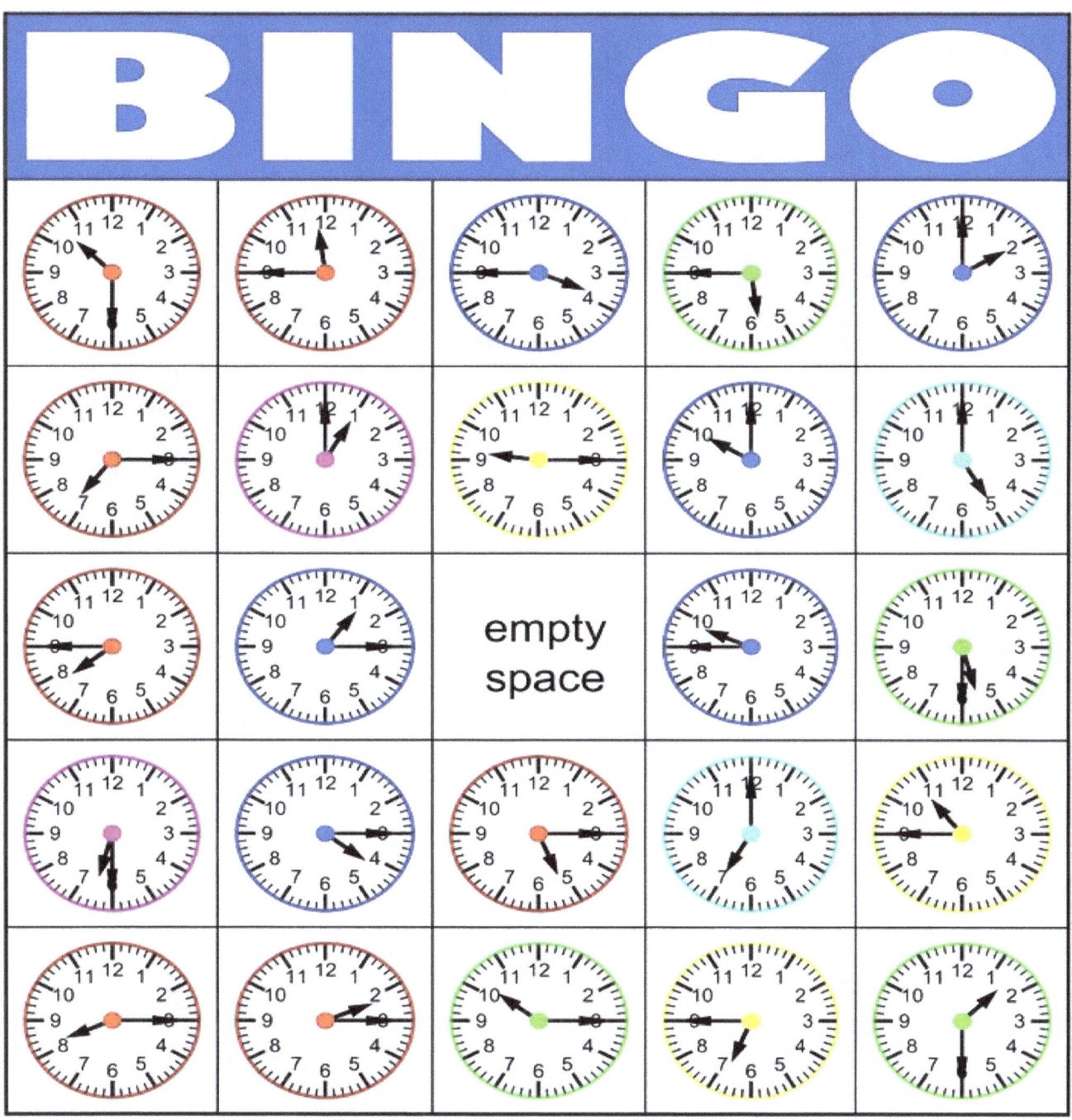

Example Only

TANGA C. ELAM, BSN, RN, MSA, BAA

Time has a wonderful way of showing us what really matters.

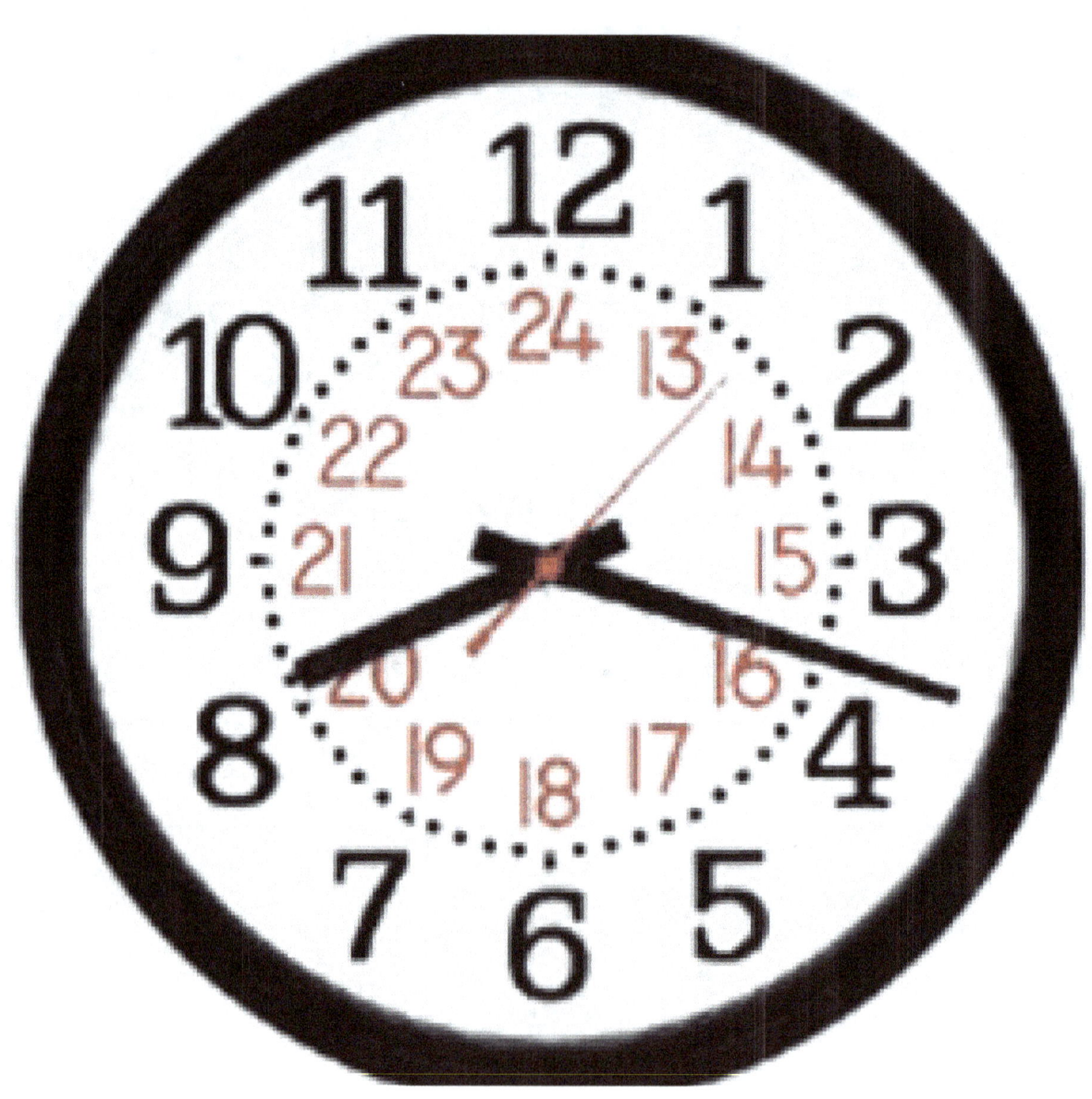

EXCELLENCE in NURSING MATH REVIEW

Duration of Time

It is 28 minutes before 5:35 pm or 1735. <u>What is the END Time?</u>

$$X = 12 + 5:35 = 1735 - 28 = 1707$$

5:07pm or 1707 is the End Time

What is the END Time?

American Eagle flight leaves from Jacksonville, Florida @ 10:37 am **AND** arrives in Washington, DC @ 2:20 pm.

- ❖ Arrival: 14:20 (2:20 pm)
- ❖ Departs: - 10:37

    Not Quite: 3:93 (93 is > 60 minutes)
                      - 40
- ❖   3:53

Here's the RULE: any minutes > 60 then subtract 40

So: The End Time is 3 hours and 53 minutes of flight time.

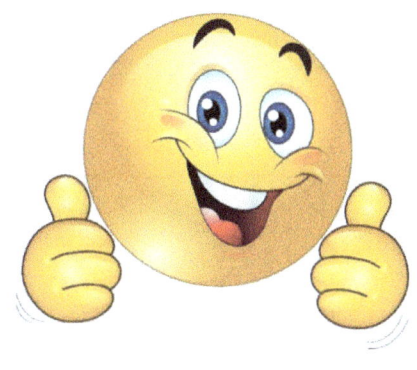

The Administration of Fluids and Drugs

Advantages of IV

- Allows direct rapid drug distribution into the bloodstream.
- It can occasionally cause minimal medication loss to the tissues.

Disadvantages of IV

- Drugs that are given IV allow less time to correct error measures. For example: A drug action is more rapid than subcutaneous (SQ) or intramuscular (IM).

Two Methods of Administration

1. Continuous

   - Replace fluid loss.
   - Maintains fluid balance.
   - Allows additional drug administration.

2. Intermittent IV

   - Piggyback—secondary sets.
   - Intermittent means meds are prescribed three to four times a day and administration in small volumes of 50 to 250 mL in D5W or NS (bags or bottles).
   - Most drugs are delivered to the patient in fifteen minutes to ninety minutes.
   - A separate tubing (secondary) is inserted into a port or primary line.
   - The difference is the shorter tubing.
   - Check drug and fluid compatibility.

IV Sets

There are various IV infusion sets produced by manufacturers. The two most common sets are 15 and 60 gtt (drip) per mL (milliliter). All micro drip sets universally deliver 60 gtt per mL. It is used for small or very precise volumes. The micro gtt is appropriate for infusions less than 100 mL / hr. The macrodrip tubing typically has:

- 10 gtts / mL
- 15 gtts / mL
- 20 gtts / mL sets

For example, if the IV rate is to infuse at 100 mL / hr or more, the macro drip sets are recommended.

It is used for larger quantities or fast rate infusion.

All IV infusions should be checked hourly to ensure the rate of infusion and assess for potential complications.

A keep vein open (KVO) purpose could be used to administer emergency drugs and to give IV drugs at scheduled hours.

Let's Get Started

Method of Calculation

D = desired dose
H = drug dose on label, container, bottle, vial, ampule, bag, or syringe
V = form and amount which drug is available in tablet / volume

D (physician ordered) x V (quantity) = X (amount to give)
H (medication available)

A zero must always be used before a decimal point.
A zero must *not* appear by itself after the decimal point.

(Note: Drop the zero following a decimal if the dose is a whole number and add a zero to the left of the decimal if the dose is a fraction.)

IV Drip Rate

- The drip factor is the drops equal 1 milliliter.
- Minutes to infuse are usually stated as hours or half hours.
- Volume to infuse divided by time to infuse = mL per hour.
- mL per hour divided by 60 = mL per minute.
- mL per min x drip factor = gtt per min.
- Round to the whole number round up if the value is >5.
- Round down if value is <5.

Formulas for calculating drip factors are:

volume in mL x drip factor = gtt / minute
time in minutes

mL / hr = **volume (mL)**
            time (hr)

EXCELLENCE in NURSING MATH REVIEW

Let's Practice

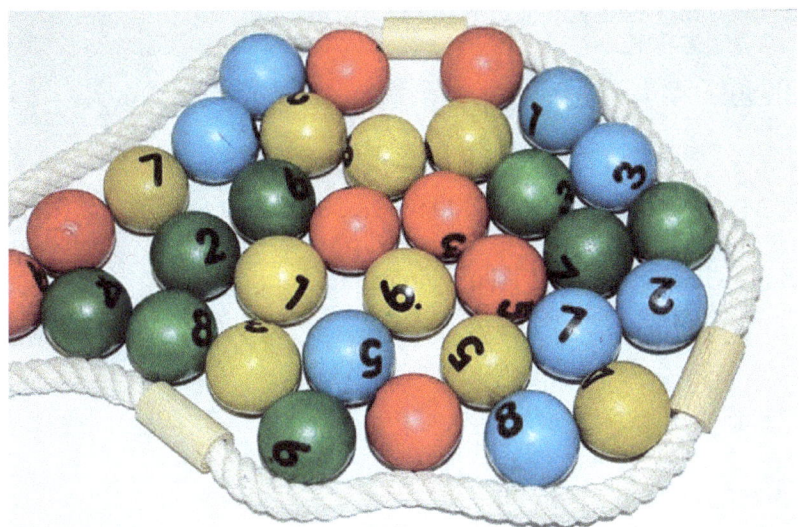

(mL / hr = gtt / min)

1. Administer Gentamycin 950 mg in 500 mL of 0.45 normal saline in 3 hours (180 minutes).
   Drop factor: 60 gtt / mL.
   Calculate the drip rate in gtt / minute.

   $$X = \frac{500 \text{ ml} \times 60 \text{ (gtt factor)}}{180 \text{ minutes} \quad \text{mL}} = \underline{\qquad} \text{ gtt / minute}$$

2. Administer Ceftriaxone (rocephin) 750 mg in 250 mL of NS in 2 hours (120 minutes).
   Drop factor: 15 gtt / mL.
   Calculate the drip rate in gtt / minute.

   $$X = \frac{250 \text{ mL} \times 15 \text{ (gtt factor)}}{120 \text{ minutes} \quad \text{mL}} = \underline{\qquad} \text{ gtt / minute}$$

3. Doctor's order: Infuse 150 mg of Amphotericin B in 500 mL NS over 4 hours and 30 minutes.
   Drop factor: 15 gtt / mL
   What flow rate (mL / hr) will you set on the IV infusion pump?

   $$X = \frac{500 \text{ mL}}{4.5 \text{ hr}} = \underline{\qquad} \text{ mL / hr}$$

4. Doctor's order: Ciprofloxacin 1 ½ L of D5NS to be infused over 9 hours.
   Drop factor: 12 gtt / mL
   What flow rate (mL / hr) will you set on the IV infusion pump?

   $$X = \frac{1500 \text{ mL}}{9 \text{ hr}} = \underline{} \text{ mL / hr}$$

5. Doctor's order: Mandol (cefamandole) 400 mg in 100 mL of D5NS to infuse IVPB 15 minutes.
   Drop factor: 10 gtt / mL.
   How many mL / hr will you set on the IV infusion pump?

   $$X = \frac{100 \text{ mL}}{0.25 \text{ hr}} = \underline{} \text{ mL / hr} \quad OR$$

   $$X = \frac{100 \text{ mL}}{15 \text{ min}} \times \frac{60 \text{ min}}{1 \text{ hr}} = \underline{} \text{ mL / hr}$$

6. Doctor's order: Infuse Dilantin (phenytoin) 1550 mL of 0.45% normal saline at 125 mL / hr
   Drop factor: 15 gtt / min.

   How many gtt / min will you regulate the IV?

   $$X = \frac{125 \text{ mL}}{60 \text{ min}} \times \frac{15 \text{ gtt}}{\text{mL}} = \underline{} \text{ gtt / min}$$

7. Doctor's order: Bivigam (intravenous immunoglobulin) 1.5 grams in 150 mL of NS to infuse IVPB in 90 minutes.
   Drop factor: 15 gtt / min

   How many gtt / min will you regulate the intravenous piggyback (IVPB)?

   $$X = \frac{150 \text{ mL}}{90 \text{ min}} \times \frac{15 \text{ gtt}}{\text{mL}} = \underline{} \text{ gtt / min}$$

8. Doctor's order: Benadryl (diphenhydramine) 3 / 4 L of D5 1 / 2 NS to infuse over 3 hours and 30 minutes.

   Drop factor: 15 gtt / mL

   How many gtt / min will you regulate the IV?

   $$X = \frac{750 \text{ mL}}{210 \text{ min}} \times \frac{15 \text{ gtt}}{\text{mL}} = \underline{} \text{ gtt / min}$$

EXCELLENCE in NURSING MATH REVIEW

9. Ordered: Keflin D5W (cephalothin) 4 g in 200 mL IVPB over 20 minutes.
   The IV tubing is 10 gtt / mL.
   Calculate the flow rate in gtt / min

   $$X = \frac{200 \text{ mL}}{20 \text{ min}} \times \frac{10 \text{ gtt}}{\text{mL}} = \underline{} \text{ gtt / min}$$

10. Ampicillin 250 mg in 150 mL IVPB over 45 minutes.
    At what rate would you set the pump in mL / hr ?

    $$X = \frac{150 \text{ mL}}{45 \text{ min}} \times \frac{60 \text{ min}}{\text{hr}} = \underline{} \text{ mL / hr}$$

11. Ordered: Vancomycin 2 grams in 250 mL IVPB is to infuse over 120 minutes.
    At what rate should the pump be set in mL / hr ?

    $$X = \frac{250 \text{ mL}}{120 \text{ min}} \times \frac{60 \text{ min}}{\text{hr}} = \underline{} \text{ mL / hr}$$

12. Etopophos (etoposide) 600 mg in 125 mL IVPB NS to run over 30 minutes.
    The tubing has a drop factor of 12 gtt / mL
    How many drops per minute should be administered?

    $$X = \frac{125 \text{ mL}}{30 \text{ min}} \times \frac{12 \text{ gtt}}{\text{mL}} = \underline{} \text{ gtt / min}$$

13. Your order reads Zosyn (tazobactam sodium) 3.5 g in 200 mL D5W IV over 2 hours.
    You have micro drip tubing.
    What drip rate will you set in gtt / min ?

    $$X = \frac{200 \text{ mL}}{2 \text{ hr}} \times \frac{1 \text{ hr}}{60 \text{ min}} \times \frac{60 \text{ gtt}}{\text{mL}} = \underline{} \text{ gtt / min}$$

14. You have 325 mL packed red blood cells (PRBCs) that you want to infuse IV over 3 hours. There is no controller available. Your blood tubing delivers 20 gtts / mL
    How many drops per minute should you set the IV pump?

    $$X = \frac{325 \text{ mL}}{3 \text{ hr}} \times \frac{20 \text{ gtt}}{\text{mL}} \times \frac{1 \text{ hr}}{60 \text{ min}} = \underline{\quad} \text{ gtt / min}$$

15. 500 mL NS with 20 meq KCL IV over 6 hrs
    Drop factor: 15 gtt / mL

    $$X = \frac{500 \text{ mL}}{6 \text{ hr}} \times \frac{15 \text{ gtt}}{\text{mL}} \times \frac{1 \text{ hr}}{60 \text{ min}} = \underline{\quad} \text{ gtt / min}$$

16. Ordered: Isotretinoin 1500 mL D5 0.45NS IV over 18 hours.
    Drop factor: 10 gtt / mL

    $$X = \frac{1500 \text{ mL}}{18 \text{ hr}} \times \frac{10 \text{ gtt}}{\text{mL}} \times \frac{1 \text{ hr}}{60 \text{ min}} = \underline{\quad} \text{ gtt / min}$$

17. Ordered: Rifampin 450 mL D5W IV over 10 hours.
    Drop factor: 15 drops / 1 mL

    $$X = \frac{450 \text{ mL}}{600 \text{ min}} \times \frac{15 \text{ gtt}}{\text{mL}} = \underline{\quad} \text{ gtt / min}$$

18. Ordered: 1000 mL of Lithium Carbonate in D10W IV over 12 hours.
    The drip set is 12 gtt / mL
    What is the rate to set the IV pump?

    $$X = \frac{1000 \text{ mL}}{720 \text{ min}} \times \frac{12 \text{ gtt}}{\text{mL}} = \underline{\quad} \text{ gtt / min}$$

EXCELLENCE in NURSING MATH REVIEW

19. Calculate in gtt / min.
    Ordered: Adriamycin (doxorubicin) 1000 mL D5NS IV in 8 hours. (60 minutes = 1 hour)
    Drop factor: 10 gtt / mL

    $$X = \frac{1000 \text{ mL} \times 10 \text{ gtt}}{480 \text{ min} \quad \text{mL}} = \underline{\qquad} \text{ gtt / min}$$

20. Ordered: Haldol (haloperidol lactate) 1000 NS IV over 16 hours = ____ mL / hr.

    $$\text{mL / hr} = \frac{1000 \text{ mL}}{16 \text{ hours}} = \underline{\qquad} \text{ mL / hr}$$

21. Ordered: Aminophylline 84 mg / hr
    Label: 1 g / 250 mL NS

    $$\text{Flow Rate} = \frac{84 \text{ mg} \times 250 \text{ mL} \times 1 \text{ g}}{1 \text{ hr} \quad 1 \text{ g} \quad 1000 \text{ mg}} = \underline{\qquad} \text{ mL / hr}$$

practice
practice
practice
practice

Answer Sheet

(mL / hr. = gtt / min)

1) 167 gtt / min
2) 31 gtt / min
3) 111.1 mL / hr
4) 167 mL / hr
5) 400 mL / hr
6) 31 gtt / min
7) 25 gtt / min
8) 54 gtt / min
9) 100 gtt / min
10) 200 mL / hr
11) 125 mL / hr
12) 50 gtt / min
13) 100 gtt / min
14) 36 gtt / min
15) 21 gtt / min
16) 14 gtt / min
17) 11 gtt / min
18) 17 gtt / min
19) 21 gtt / min
20) 62.5 mL / hr
21) 21 mL / hr

IV Fractional Hours

Additional information: How long will it take to complete an IV medication on the pump? Fractional hours are necessary for practice to get the accurate drug amount.

Formula: Rate = $\frac{\text{Time or Volume}}{\text{Rate}}$ = Infusion Time Flow

practice
practice
practice
practice

4. Vfend (voriconazole) 1000 mL of D5W IV infusing @ 80 mL / hr

   $\frac{1000 \text{ mL} \times 1 \text{ hr}}{80 \text{ mL}}$ = 12.5 hrs or 12 hrs and 30 min infusing time

   $\frac{12 \text{ hr and } 0.5 \text{ hr (fractional hrs)} \times 60 \text{ min}}{1 \text{ hr}}$ = 30 min

5. Cisplatin IV of 750 mL in LR ordered @ rate of 90 mL / hr

   $\frac{750 \text{ mL} \times 1 \text{ hr}}{90 \text{ mL}}$ = 8.3 hrs or 8 hrs and 18 min infusing time

   $\frac{8 \text{ hrs and } 0.3 \text{ hr (fractional hrs.)} \times 60 \text{ min}}{1 \text{ hr}}$ = 18 min

6. Mucomyst (acetylcysteine) of 500 mL 0.45NS ordered @ rate of 55 mL / hr

   $\frac{500 \text{ mL} \times 1 \text{ hr}}{55 \text{ mL}}$ = 9.09 hrs or 9 hrs and 5 min infusing time

   9 hrs and 0.09 hr (fractional hrs) x 60 min = 5.4 min

IV Time Remaining

There are times when the IV infusion via the pump will have time remaining to completion.

Formula: Time Remaining = $\dfrac{\text{current volume (mL)}}{\text{pump setting (mL)}}$

1. How much longer will this infusion have to continue?

   Pt received 150 mL D10W IV
   Current volume of 100 mL of D10W IV Pump setting @ 30mL / hr

   HINT: 150 ml–100 ml = 50 mL

   Time remaining = $\dfrac{50 \text{ mL}}{30 \text{ mL / hr}}$ = 1.66 hr

   Minutes = 60 min x 0.66 = 39.6 min = 40 min Total time remaining = 1 hr and 40 min

2. What is time remaining on the IV pump?

   Pt received 350 mL of D5 NS IV Current volume of 50 mL of D5NS IV Pump setting @ 40 mL / hr

   Remaining = $\dfrac{300 \text{ mL}}{40 \text{ mL / hr}}$ = 7.5 hours

   Minutes = 60 min x 0.5 = 30 min

   Total time remaining = 7 hr and 30 min

3. What is the time remaining on the IV pump?

   Pt received 1520 mL of LR IV Current
   volume of 625 mL of LR IV Pump
   setting @ 65 mL / hr

   Time remaining = $\dfrac{895 \text{ mL}}{65 \text{ mL / hr}}$ = 13.8 hrs

   Minutes = 60 min x 0.8 = 48 min
   Total time remaining = 13 hrs and 48 min

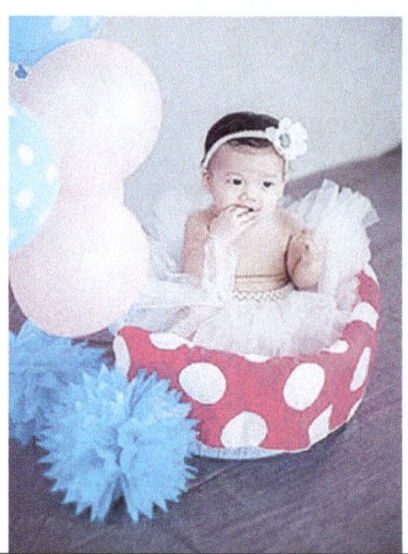

Pediatric Dosages

The dose of medication for a pediatric client *must be* carefully calculated based on weight per kilogram (mg / kg) or body surface area (BSA) (mg / m²).

Converting pounds to kilograms (1 kg = 2.2 lb) is necessary for safe medication administration. Even a small discrepancy can endanger the youngest client.

Small children who are administered medications are at risk for overdose, toxic reactions, and even death.

At the start of birth to one year of age, pediatrics will maintain a greater percentage of body water. From age one to twelve years of age, a child can metabolize drugs more readily than adults. This is because of their immature physiological processes such as absorption, distribution, metabolism, and excretion.

Safe Pediatric Dosages

Calculated by two formulas:

- Body weight which is usually measured in mg per kg and mcg per kg
- Body surface area (BSA) is measured in (m squared) m2

Pediatric Formula: Weight = 3 (age) +7

This formula can be used over a larger age range (from one year to puberty) and allows a safe and more accurate estimate of the weight of children today according to Emerg Med J. (2012).

- 1 kg = 2.2 pounds (lb)
- Convert child's pounds to kilograms (kg) by dividing 2.2

When converting pounds to kilograms, round kilogram weight (wgt.) to one decimal place (tenths)

Approximate Weight Per Age
- Newborn: 4 kg
- 6 months: 7 kg
- 1 year: 10 kg
- 2–3 years: 12–14 kg
- 4–5 years: 16–18 kg
- 6–8 years: 20–26 kg
- 8–10 years: 26–32 kg
- 10–14 years: 32–50 kg
- 14 years: > 50 kg

Notes

- ✓ The maximum quantity of medication should be allowed 24 hours before administrating medication to a child.
- ✓ Medication tablets and / or capsules are often supplied in milligrams (mg).
- ✓ Antibiotics are usually supplied in grams (g), milligrams (mg), or units.
- ✓ Micrograms (mcg) are used primarily in pediatrics and intensive care units.

TANGA C. ELAM, BSN, RN, MSA, BAA

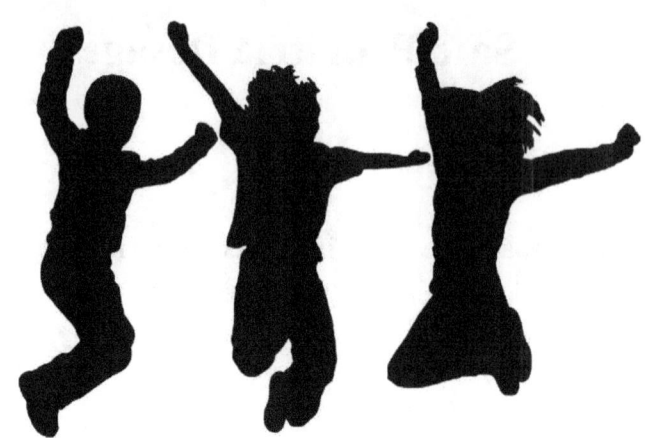

Pediatric Practice Problems

Dose = <u>orders per kg x ped's wgt (kg) x quantity</u>
dose on hand

1. Ordered: Romazicon 15 mcg / kg Available: flumazenil 50 mcg / mL
   Pediatrics wt. of 55 lb = (25 kg)
   How many mL will the client receive?

   $$X = \frac{15 \text{ mcg} \times 25 \text{ kg} \times 1 \text{ mL}}{1 \text{ kg} \times 50 \text{ mcg}} = \underline{\quad} \text{ mL}$$

2. Ordered: Reglan 2.8 mg / kg by mouth (po) (3x day) tid
   Available: metoclopramide 15.5 mg capsules (caps)
   Child's wt. of 37 lbs = 16.8 kg
   How many caps will a 37 lb child receive per dose?

   $$A = 2.8 \text{ mg} / \text{kg} \times 16.8 \text{ kg} = 47 \text{ mg (per dose)}$$
   $$B = \frac{47 \text{ mg} \times 1 \text{ cap}}{15.5 \text{ mg}} = \underline{\quad} \text{ caps}$$

EXCELLENCE in NURSING MATH REVIEW

3. Ordered: Diflucan 9.2 mg / kg IM every 8 hrs
   Available: fluconazole 0.75 g / mL   (1 g = 1000 mg)
   Child's wt. of 124 lbs = 56.4 kg
   How many mL will a 124 lb child receive / dose?

   $$A = 9.2 \text{ mg/kg} \times 56.4 \text{ kg} = 518.9 \text{ mg}$$
   $$B = \frac{518.9 \text{ mg} \times 1 \text{ mL}}{750 \text{ mg}} = \underline{\quad} \text{ mL}$$

4. Order: Cogentin 3.25 mg / lb IM every 12 hr
   Available: benztropine 0.55 g / 4.3 mL
   Child's wt. of 38 kg = 83.6 lbs
   How many mL will a 38 kg child receive per day?

   $$A = 3.25 \text{ mg/lbs} \times 83.6 \text{ lbs} = 271.7 \text{ mg}$$
   $$B = \frac{271.7 \text{ mg} \times 4.3 \text{ mL}}{550} = \underline{\quad} \text{ mL} \times 2 = \underline{\quad} \text{ mL}$$

5. Give: Adderall 75 mg / kg / day po tid
   This child weighs: 35.8 kg
   Label: amphetamine & dextroamphetamine is in an oral suspension of 150 mg / 2 mL
   How many mL would be administered per dose?

   $$A = 75 \text{ mg/kg} \times 35.8 \text{ kg} = 2685 \text{ mg}$$
   $$B = \frac{2685 \text{ mg} \times 2 \text{ mL}}{150} = \underline{\quad} \text{ mL per dose}$$

6. Give Ceclor 55 mg / kg / day po in 4 divided doses
   Patient weighs 76 pounds
   This 95 mL stock medication is labeled cefaclor of 155 mg / mL.
   How many mL would you administer per dose?

   $$A = 55 \text{ mg/kg/day} \times 34.5 \text{ kg} = 1897.5 \text{ mg/day} \div 4 \text{ doses} = \underline{\quad} \text{ mg per dose}$$
   $$B = \frac{474 \text{ mg} \times 1 \text{ mL} / 4 \text{ doses}}{155 \text{ mg}} = \underline{\quad} \text{ mL}$$

7. Administer: Lamictal (lamotrigine) is 10 mg / kg / day in divided doses every 6 hours.
   Child's weight is 84 pounds = (38.2 kg)
   How many mg per dose will this child receive?

   $$X = 10 \text{ mg} \times 38.2 \text{ kg} / 4 \text{ doses} = \rule{1cm}{0.15mm} \text{ mg every 6 hrs}$$

8. An 11-year-old child weighs 52 kg

   Recommended daily dose of Bactrim (sulfamethoxazole & trimethoprim) is 340 - 500 mg / kg / day po which is divided every 8 hours.

   What's the maximum daily dose that this child can receive per day?

   $$X_a = 340 \text{ mg} \times 52 \text{ kg} / \text{day} = \text{not needed in equation}$$
   $$X_b = 500 \text{ mg} \times 52 \text{ kg} / \text{day} = \rule{1cm}{0.15mm} \text{ mg per day}$$

9. A safe maintenance dose of Risperdal (risperidone) is 0.76 mg / kg / hour.
   It is supplied as 200 mg / 150 mL.
   The patient is 140 pounds and is receiving 10 mL / hour.

   Is the dose safe?   Yes or No

   First, let's compare a safe dose to the patient's dose. You will need to configure two separate calculations:

   $$X_a = \frac{0.76 \text{ mg} \times 1 \text{ kg} \times 140 \text{ lb}}{\text{kg / hr} \quad\quad 2.2 \text{ lb}} = \rule{1cm}{0.15mm} \text{ mg / hr}$$

   $$X_b = \frac{10 \text{ mL} \times 200 \text{ mg}}{\text{hr} \quad\quad 150 \text{ mL}} = \rule{1cm}{0.15mm} \text{ mg / hr}$$

   Yes, this is a safe dose but not therapeutic.

practice
practice
practice
practice

EXCELLENCE in NURSING MATH REVIEW

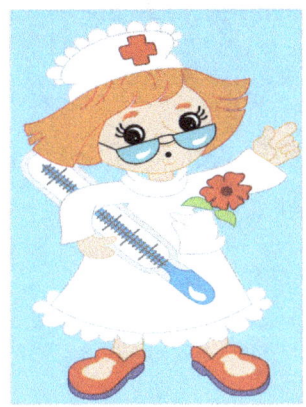

Pediatric Multiple Dose per Day

Dose / Day = orders / kg x ped's wgt (kg) x quantity = mL med
                                on hand

Then next dose = dose / day = mL
                ordered # of doses

10. Ordered Paxil: 75 mg / kg / day po every 8 hours
    Label is paroxetine: 150 mg / mL

    Child's wt. is 48 lb = ▩ kg

    a. dose / day = 75 mg x 21.8 kg x mL = ▩ mL / day
                     150 mg   x   1 kg

    b. dose = 10.9 mL   = ▩ mL / 24 hrs   (hint: every 8 hr x 3 = 24 hrs)
              3 doses ordered

11. Ordered Xanax: 150 mcg / kg / day po every 6 hours
    Available is alprazolam: 3000 mcg / mL

    Client's wt. is 78 lb = (▩ kg)   remember 1kg = 2.2 lb

    A) dose / day = 150 mcg x 35.5 kg x mL = ▩ mL / day
                      3000 mcg   x   1 kg

    B) dose / 24 hr = 1.8 mL = ▩ mL / 24 hr   (hint: every 6 hr x 4 = 24 hr)
                       4 doses

12. Prescribed Librium: 30 mg / kg / day every 4 hours
    Labeled: chlordiazepoxide hydrochloride: 125 mg / 5 mL

    Ped's wt. is 42 lb (kg)

    A)   dose / day = $\dfrac{30 \text{ mg} \times 19.1 \text{ kg} \times 5 \text{ mL}}{125 \text{ mg} \times 1 \text{ kg}}$ =   mL / day

    B)   dose / 24 hr = $\dfrac{22.9 \text{ mL}}{6 \text{ doses}}$ =   mL / 24 hr

13. Ordered: Phenergan 1.3 mg / kg

    Child weight is 84.6 lb (kg)
    On hand is promethazine: 175 mg / 3 mL

    X = $\dfrac{1.3 \text{ mg} \times 38.5 \text{ kg} \times 3 \text{ mL}}{175 \text{ mg} \times 1 \text{ kg}}$ =   mL

EXCELLENCE in NURSING MATH REVIEW

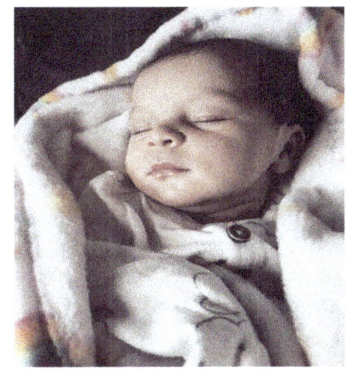

Pharmacy Pediatric Dosing Formulas

- **Fred's rule**: $\dfrac{\text{Age in months} \times \text{adult dose}}{150}$ = child's dose

- **Young's rule**: $\dfrac{\text{Age of child in years} \times \text{adult dose}}{(\text{age of child in yrs} + 12)}$ = child's dose

- **Clark's rule**: $\dfrac{\text{Child's weight in pounds} \times \text{adult dose}}{150}$ = child's dose

14. *(FR)* How much Carafate should a 7-month-old infant receive po if the adult dose is 250 mg?

    How many mL will the infant receive if the available sucralfate medication is 100 mg / 2.5 mL?

    $X = \dfrac{7 \times 250 \text{ mg}}{150} = \underline{}$ mg

    $X = \dfrac{11.7 \text{ mg} \times 2.5 \text{ mL}}{100 \text{ mg}} = \underline{}$ mL

15. **(YR)** How many mg of Enulose will a 13-year-old child receive po if the adult dose is 8 mg?

    The lactulose medication is labeled as 3mg / 7 mL

    How much will this child receive?

    X = 13 x 8 mg = 104 = ▒ mg / dose
        (13 + 12)   25

    X = 4.2 mg x 7 mL = ▒ mL
         3 mg

16. **(CR)** How many mg of Neurontin will a 72-lb child receive po if the adult dose is 1250 mg?

    The gabapentin is labeled as 750 mg / 10 mL

    How many mL will the child receive?

    X = 72 x 1250 mg = ▒ mg / dose
           150

    X = 600 mg x 10 mL = ▒ mL
          750 mg

practice
practice
practice
practice

EXCELLENCE in NURSING MATH REVIEW

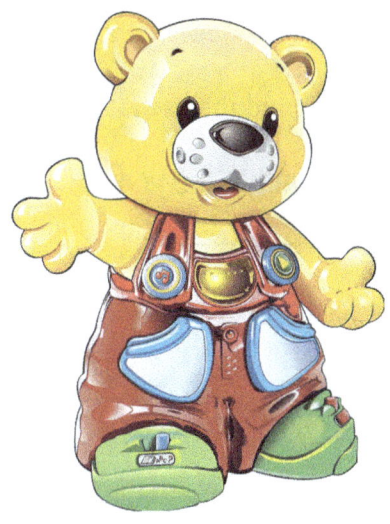

BSA Formula

BSA Formula: $\sqrt{\dfrac{\text{child's BSA (m}^2\text{) x adult dose}}{1.73 \text{ m}^2}}$ = child's dose

17. Give Biaxin to a child whose BSA is 0.45 m². The usual adult dose is 500 mg.

    Clarithromycin is available in an oral suspension.

    The bottle is labeled 125 mg / 1.5 mL.

    How many mL would you give per dose?

    $X = \sqrt{\dfrac{0.45 \text{ m}^2 \text{ x } 500 \text{ mg}}{1.73 \text{ m}^2}}$ = ____ mg → $\dfrac{132.35 \text{ mg x } 1.5 \text{ mL}}{125 \text{ mg}}$ = ____ mL

18. Give Cymbalta to a child whose BSA is 2.2 m². The usual adult dose is 65 mg.

    How many milligrams of duloxetine would you administer PO for the dose?

    $X = \sqrt{\dfrac{2.2 \text{ m}^2 \text{ x } 65 \text{ mg}}{1.73 \text{ m}^2}}$ = ____ mg

19. The child has a BSA of 0.42 m²

    The prescribed Pradaxa medication for adult dose is 50 mg

    How much dabigatran should the child receive PO?

    $$BSA = \sqrt{\frac{0.42\ m^2 \times 50\ mg}{1.73\ m^2}} = \sqrt{0.2428 \times 50\ mg} = 3.48\ mg$$

20. A client's height of 110 cm. The weight is 20.5 kg.

    The Aricept medication of an adult dose is 42 mg.

    What mg dose of donepezil should this patient receive po?

    $$BSA = \sqrt{\frac{110\ cm \times 20.5\ kg}{3600}} = \sqrt{\frac{2255}{3600}} = \sqrt{0.63} = 0.79\ m^2$$

    $$\text{Child dose} = \sqrt{\frac{0.79\ m^2 \times 42\ mg}{1.73\ m^2}} = 4.38\ mg$$

21. What is the required dose for a child with a BSA of 0.52 m² ?

    The prescribed Zoloft (sertraline) medication dose is 25 mg / m² .

    $X = 0.52\ m^2 \times 25\ mg/m^2 = 13\ mg$

Pediatric Answer Sheet

1) 7.5

2) 3

3) 0.7

4) 2.1 / 4.2

5) 35.8

6) 0.8

7) 95.5

8) 26,000

9) 48.4 / 13.3 / yes

10) 10.9 / 3.6

11) 1.8 / 0.5

12) 22.9 / 3.8

13) 0.9

14) 11.7 / 0.3

15) 4.2 / 9.8

16) 600 / 8

17) 1.6

18) 1.6

19) 1.3 / 1.14 / 57

20) 1.3

21) 13

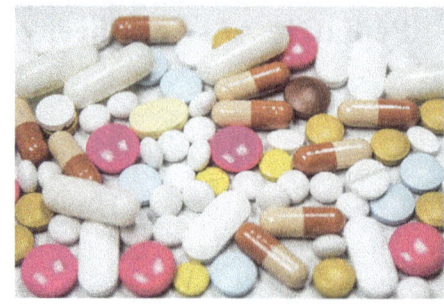

At times, you may be required to calculate adult drug dosages using BSA (body surface area).

The formulas to calculate BSA are:

$$BSA\ (m^2) = \sqrt{\frac{hgt\ (in) \times wgt\ (lb)}{3131}} \quad \text{(household)}$$

$$BSA\ (m^2) = \sqrt{\frac{height\ (cm) \times weight\ (kg)}{3600}} \quad \text{(metric)}$$

1. What is the BSA in m² of a male weight the height of 6 feet 2 inches? His weight is 197 lbs.

   A) 6 ft x 12 in +2 = 74 in

   B) $\sqrt{\frac{74 \times 197}{3131}} = \sqrt{4.65} = $ ▢ m²

   C) BSA = ▢ m²

2. What is the BSA in m² of a female patient with a height of 5'6" and a weight of 170 lbs.

   A) 5 ft x 12 in + 6 = ▢ in

   B) $\sqrt{\frac{66\ ins \times 170}{3131}} = \sqrt{3.58} = $ ▢ m²

   C) BSA = ▢ m²

3. What is the BSA in m² of a client with a height of 185 cm and weight of 98 kg?

   BSA = $\sqrt{\frac{185 \times 95}{3600}} = \sqrt{4.88} = $ ▢ m²

EXCELLENCE in NURSING MATH REVIEW

4. What is the BSA in m² of a patient with a height of 110 cm and weight of 67 kg?

$$BSA = \sqrt{\frac{110 \times 67}{3600}} = \sqrt{2.04} = \underline{} \ m^2$$

5. The patient's height is 92 cm, and the weight is 15.8 kg.

   The prescribed Solu-Cortef (hydrocortisone) medication is 130 mg / m².

   What should this patient receive in mg?

$$BSA = \sqrt{\frac{92 \times 15.8}{3600}} = \sqrt{\frac{1454}{3600}} = \sqrt{0.40} = \underline{} \ m^2 = 130 \ mg \times 0.64 = \underline{} \ mg$$

(BSA (m²)) Answer Sheet

1) 2.16

2) 1.89

3) 2.21

4) 1.43

5) 83.2

Metric Units

Converting metric units: This is my favorite formula because it's easy to remember.

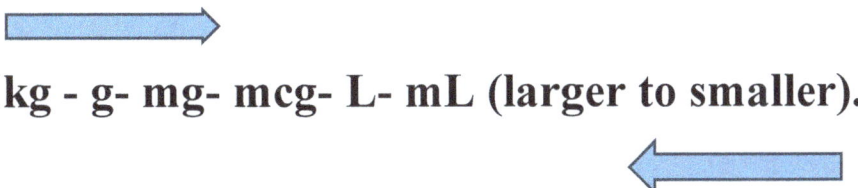

kg - g- mg- mcg- L- mL (larger to smaller).

There are times when the unit of the medication order will be different from the unit of the medication label. So, with the above formula, if you multiply by 1000, move to the right when converting from larger to smaller values.

Or, moving from smaller to larger value then divide by 1000. Moving three decimal points in either direction is not necessary. Just from left to right and right to left is the main point.

TRUST THE PROCESS®

The simplest way to perform conversions involving metric quantities is to memorize the equivalents, which can save lives.

Metric System Used in Dose Calculation

- Weight is most used in mcg, mg and gram
- Liter and milliliter measures volume
- Meter measures length

Commonly Used Metric Equivalences for Weight

- **1 kg = 2.2 lbs = 1,000 g**
- **1 g = 1,000 mg**
- **1 mg = 1,000 mcg**
- **1 liter = 1,000 mL**
- **1 mL = 1 cc**
- ***1 hr = 60 minutes can be used interchangeably**

(MNEMONIC)

King   Henry   Died   By   Drinking   Chocolate   Milk

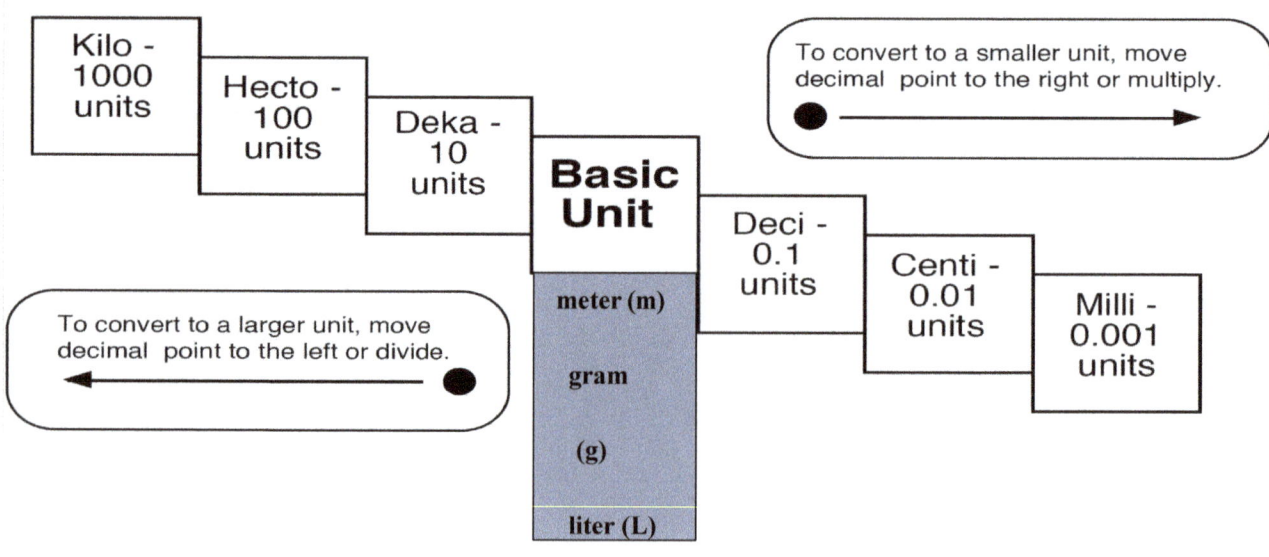

EXCELLENCE in NURSING MATH REVIEW

Let's Practice with Metric Units

1. Order: Tylenol supp 2 g per rectum (pr) every 12 hr as needed (prn).
   Available: acetaminophen suppository (supp) 325 mg (scored)
   How many supp will you administer?

   $$1 \text{ g} = 1000 \text{ mg}$$

   $$X = \frac{2 \text{ g} \times 1000 \text{ mg} \times 1 \text{ supp}}{325 \text{ mg} \quad 1 \text{ g}} = \underline{} \text{ supp}$$

2. Order: Urecholine 750 mg po (by mouth) *pc* (after meal)
   Available: bethanechol chloride 1 g tablet (scored tab)
   How many tabs will you administer per day?

   $$1 \text{ g} = 1000 \text{ mg}$$

   $$X = \frac{750 \text{ mg} \times 1 \text{ g} \times 3 \text{ meals} \times 1 \text{ tab}}{1 \text{ g} \quad 1000 \text{ mg}} = \underline{} \text{ tabs}$$

3. Order: Loxitane 75 mcg po daily
   Available: loxapine 0.3 mg tab (scored)
   How many tabs will you administer?

   $$1 \text{ mg} = 1000 \text{ mcg}$$

   $$X = \frac{75 \text{ mcg} \times 1 \text{ mg} \times 1 \text{ tab}}{0.3 \text{ mg} \quad 1000 \text{ mcg}} = \underline{} \text{ tab}$$

4. Order: Streptomycin 3.25 mg / lb. IM every 18 hours
   Available: streptomycin 0.15 g / 5.3 mL
   How many mL will you administer a 79 kg patient / 8 hr ?

   79 kg = 173.8 lbs
   3.25 mg / lbs x 173.8 lbs = ____ mg

   $$X = \frac{564.9 \text{ mg} \times 1 \text{ g}}{0.15 \text{ g} \quad 1000 \text{ mg}} \times 5.3 \text{ mL} = \underline{} \text{ mL}$$

Household Measurements

- 1 g = gr (grain) xv (15)
- gr i = 60 mg or 65 mg (in select instances)
- 1 t (teaspoon) = 5 mL (milliliter) = 60 gtt
- 1 T (tablespoon) = 3 t = 15 mL = ½ fluid ounce
- 1 fluid ounce = 30 mL = 2 T = 6 t
- 1 cup (glass) = 240 mL = 8 fluid ounce
- 1 lb. (pound) = 16 ounces
- 1 inch = 2.54 cm

5. The pre-op patient ordered Atropine 1 / 250 gr IV.
   The vial contains Atropine 0.8 mg in 1 mL

   How much will you give?

   *1gr = 60 mg

   $$Xa = \frac{1/250 \text{ gr} \times 60 \text{ mg}}{1 \text{ gr}} = \underline{} \text{ mg}$$

   $$Xb = \frac{0.24 \text{ mg} \times 1 \text{ mL}}{0.8 \text{ mg}} = \underline{} \text{ mL}$$

6. Ordered codeine 1 / 4 gr IM every 2 hours prn.
   On hand codeine 1 / 2 gr per mL

   What is the correct dose?

   $$X = \frac{1/4 \text{ gr} \times 1 \text{ mL}}{1/2 \text{ gr}} = \underline{} \text{ mL}$$

EXCELLENCE in NURSING MATH REVIEW

7. Ordered: Ecotrin gr V po.
   Available: aspirin 300 mg tablet

   How many tablets would you administer?

   Note: 1 gr = 60 mg

   X = 5 gr x 60 mg = 300 mg / 300 mg tab = ▒ tablet
         1 gr

8. A home care patient must restrict fluid intake to 4 L every 48 hours.
   He has household measuring cups.

   How many cups may he drink daily and not exceed the 4L limit?

   X = 4 L x 1000 mL x 1 cup / 2 days = ▒ cups per 24 hours
         1 L   240 mL

9. You are providing home care for a patient who needs 45 mL of Maalox (magnesium / aluminum hydroxide) po.

   The client has only standard measuring spoons in the house.

   How do you instruct the client to take the po dose?

   X = 45 mL x 1 tbsp = ▒ tbsp
             15 mL

10. Synthroid (levothyroxine) is ordered @ 125 mcg PO daily.
    On hand there is 0.1 mg tablets (scored).

    _____many tabs per day?

    ❖   1 mg = 1000 mcg

    X = 125 mcg x 1 mg   x 1 tab = ▒ tabs
          1000 mcg 0.1 mg

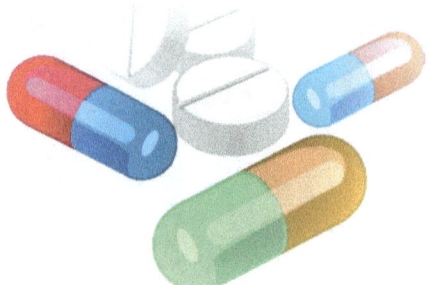

11. Capoten 250 mcg PO per day is ordered. This med is supplied as 0.045 mg tablets. The patient weighs 186 pounds. A safe dose of captopril is 3.5 mcg / kg / day.

    How many tablets should the patient take daily?

    Is this safe to administer? Yes   or   No

    $$X = \frac{250 \text{ mcg}}{1000 \text{ mcg}} \times \frac{1 \text{ mg}}{0.045 \text{ mg}} \times \text{tab} = \boxed{} \text{ tabs daily}$$

    $$X = \frac{250 \text{ mcg} \times 2.2 \text{ lbs}}{186 \text{ lbs} \quad \text{kg}} = \boxed{} \text{ mcg / kg}$$

    *Yes, this dose is safe because 3 mcg / kg is less than 3.5 mcg / kg / day.

12. You have an order for 250 mg Procrit (epoetin alfa) IVPB every 8 hours for a patient who weighs 210 lbs. You know that you can safely administer up to 50 mg / kg / day.

    Is the order safe? Yes or No

    $$X = \frac{250 \text{ mg} \times 3 \text{ doses} \times 2.2 \text{ lbs}}{210 \text{ lbs} \quad \text{day} \quad 1 \text{ kg}} = \boxed{} \text{ mg / kg / day}$$

    Yes, the order is safe because 7.8 mg / kg is less than the safe dose of 50 mg / **kg**

13. A patient is taking Zyloprim (allopurinol) 325 mg, 2 tablets PO every 12 hrs.

    How many grams is the patient receiving in 24 hours?

    $$X = \frac{325 \text{ mg} \times 2 \text{ tabs} \times 2 \text{ doses} \times 1 \text{ g}}{\text{tab} \quad \text{dose} \quad \text{day} \quad 1000 \text{ mg}} = \boxed{} \text{ g}$$

EXCELLENCE in NURSING MATH REVIEW

Metric Units Answer Sheet

1) 6

2) 2.25

3) 0.25

4) 20

5) 0.3

6) 0.5

7) 1

8) 8.3

9) 3

10) 1.25

11) 5.5 / 3

12) 7.8

13) 1.3

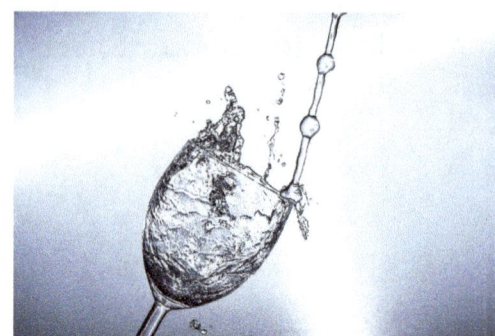
8x8: Rule or Myth?

Drinking eight 8-ounce glasses of water every day would equate to a total of sixty-four fluid ounces or 1.9 liters of fluid.

A 2009 Scientific American article suggests that the 8x8 rule was originally developed because the Food and Nutrition Board once suggested that people consume 1 milliliter of water for every calorie of food consumed, which equates to about sixty-four ounces on a 1,900-calorie-per-day diet.

But while the 8x8 idea might not actually be based on scientific evidence, it is not a bad rule to include in your lifestyle. It is an effortless way to remember to drink plenty of water throughout the day.

However, it should be imperative to consider age, gender, health status, environment, and lifestyle to determine an individual's proper daily fluid intake.

The National Academies of Sciences, Engineering, and Medicine determined that an adequate daily fluid intake is:

- About 15.5 cups (3.7 liters) of fluids for men
- About 11.5 cups (2.7 liters) of fluids a day for women

These recommendations cover fluids from water, other beverages, and food. About 20 percent of daily fluid intake usually comes from food and the rest from drinks.

However, pregnant women should aim for 3 liters per day, and lactating women need 3.8 liters per day. The daily adequate intake of water is lower before the age of 18.

From birth to 12 months of age, infants need just 0.7 to 0.8 liters per day, which is easily achieved through breast milk alone.

The daily intake increases to 1.3 liters from age 1 to 3 and 1.7 liters from age 4 to 8.

Males then need 2.4 to 3.3 liters per day until the age of eighteen, while females need just 2.1 to 2.3 liters per day until they reach adulthood.

Recording Daily Intake

This fluid can come from all forms of drinks and even moisture from food, but it is only a guideline. Exercising or any other form of physical exertion will use up your water supplies and should be replenished whenever you feel thirsty.

Recording daily intake can include oral intake, tube feedings, intravenous fluids, medications, total parenteral nutrition, lipids, blood products, dialysis fluids, and flushes.

Most institutions require the clinician to document the input and output every one to two hours. Some of the critical care units require strict measurements, for which means every milliliter of fluid should be accounted.

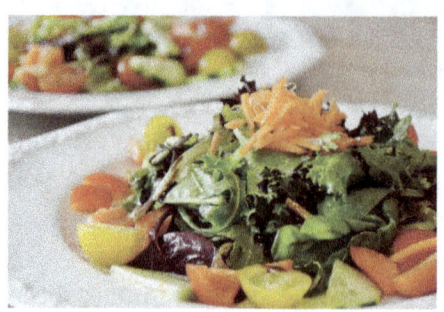

1. Record daily liquid intake and output for client with renal failure.

    - 32 ounces water
    - 4 ounces orange juice
    - 1 pint blueberry yogurt
    - 1.5 L Normal Saline IV

    Note: 1 oz = 30 mL
         1 pint = 500 mL
         1 L = 1000 mL

    Calculate the total input for this client.

    X = 36 oz x 30 mL = 1080 mL
        1 pint yogurt = 500 mL
        1.5 L fluids = 1500 mL

    Total Intake = _____ mL daily

EXCELLENCE in NURSING MATH REVIEW

2. Your patient has had the following intake:

   - 3 ½ cups of coffee
   - 8 oz of carrot juice
   - 2 qt of skim milk
   - 360 mL of sparkling water
   - 2 ¼ L of D5NS IV and 2 oz of grits

   What will you record as the total intake in mL for this patient?

   Note: 1 cup = 240 mL
   　　　1 qt = 1000 mL
   　　　1 oz = 30 mL

   X = 3.5 cups x 240 mL = 840 mL
   　　8 oz x 30 mL = 240 mL
   　　2 qt x 1000 mL = 2000 mL
   　　sparkling water = 360 mL
   　　D5NS IV = 2250 mL

   Total Intake = _____ mL

   (Grits are not liquid at room temperature, which is not included when calculating intake.)

Calculate Daily Output

Calculating a patient's 12-hour output will require you to record all fluids that are excreted or withdrawn from the patient. This includes urine, liquid stool, drainage from drains or chest tubes, and critical areas of blood.

Basically, you will check all urine bags, drains, and collection canisters every one to two hours. If a patient uses diapers or voids on the protective pad, you can weigh a dry one and then weigh the soiled one subtract the standard weight to calculate the output.

Estimate the patient's 12-hour (7:00 a.m-7:00 p.m.) output

0800–urine 100 mL
0800–suction canister 50 mL
0800 –chest tube 35 mL

1000–urine 150 mL
1000–chest tube 25 mL

1200–urine 120 mL
1200–suction canister 30 mL
1200–chest tube 15 mL

1400–urine 130 mL
1400–chest tube 10 mL

1600–urine 120 mL
1600–suction canister 20 mL 1600–
chest tube 10 mL

1800–urine 150 mL
1800–chest tube 10 mL

Total = urine 770 + canister 100 + chest tube 105 =

How many milliliters should you record as output?

What is the difference between the patient's intake and output above?

EXCELLENCE in NURSING MATH REVIEW

Overload Versus Dehydration

Average daily oral intake for an adult is 1200–1500 mL, and the output should be equivalent to the intake. If the difference is less than 500 mL, then the ratio is adequate.

If the difference of the total intake and total output is a positive number, then the body has retained fluids.

The opposite is when a negative number of differences incurs that more fluids have been lost while the patient is at risk for dehydration.

A patient's current weight plays a factor in determining the plan of care.

Examples:

1. Total Intake = 1430 mL
   Total Output = 950 mL
   Difference =

   Is this patient at risk for fluid overload or dehydration? _____

2. Total Intake = 2312 mL
   Total Output = 3780 mL
   Difference =

   Is this patient at risk for fluid overload or dehydration? _____

3. Total Intake = 5557mL
   Total Output = 2762 mL
   Difference =

   Is this patient at risk for fluid overload or dehydration? _____

TANGA C. ELAM, BSN, RN, MSA, BAA

Answer Sheet

(Daily Intake and Output)

Intake	Output	Differences between I & O
3080	975	480 No < 500 mL
5690		1468 Dehydration
		2795 Overload

EXCELLENCE in NURSING MATH REVIEW

Practice makes Progress

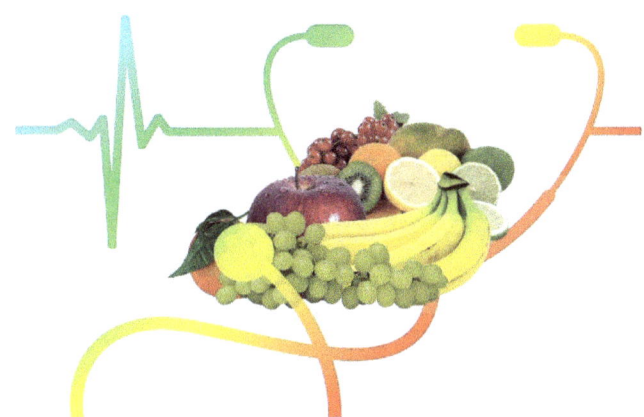

Reconstitution of Meds

1. Order: Cleocin Oral Susp 900 mg po bid.
   Directions for mixing: Add 125 mL of water and shake vigorously.
   Each 3.5 mL will contain 300 mg of clindamycin.

   How many teaspoons of Cleocin will you administer?

   $$1\ tsp = 5\ mL$$

   $$X_a = \frac{900\ mg}{300\ mg} \times 3.5\ mL = \underline{\quad}\ mL$$

   $$X_b = \underline{\quad}\ mL \times \frac{1\ tsp}{5\ mL} = \underline{\quad}\ tsp$$

2. Order: Azulfidine Oral Suspension 1500 mg every 8 hours
   Directions for mixing: Add 100 mL of water and shake well.
   Each tablespoon will yield 2.5 g of sulfasalazine.

   How many mL will you give?

   $$1\ tbsp = 15\ mL$$

   $$X = \frac{1500\ mg}{2.5\ g} \cdot \frac{1\ g}{1000\ mg} \times 15\ mL = \underline{\quad}\ mL$$

3. Order: Reclast 0.5 mg IV bolus 4x daily (QID)
   Instructions: Constitute zoledronic acid to 2000 micrograms / 4.3 mL with 4.8mL of 5% dextrose water for injection.

   How many mL will you administer?

   $$1 \text{ mg} = 1000 \text{ mcg}$$

   $$X = \frac{0.5 \text{ mg} \times 1000 \text{ mcg} \times 4.3 \text{ mL}}{2000 \text{ mcg} \quad 1 \text{ mg}} = \underline{} \text{ mL}$$

4. Order: Tazidime 0.7 g IM daily
   Reconstitution: For IM solution, add 2.5 mL of diluent. Shake to dissolve ceftazidime. Provides an approximate volume of 1.8 mL (260 mg / mL).

   How many milliliters will you give?

   $$1 \text{ g} = 1000 \text{ mg}$$

   $$X = \frac{0.7 \text{ g} \times 1000 \text{ mg} \times 1 \text{ mL}}{260 \text{ mg} \quad 1 \text{ g}} = \underline{} \text{ mL}$$

5. Administer Famvir (famciclovir): 0.25 g IV QID
   Reconstitute with 9 mL of sterile water = 400 mg / 2 mL

   $$X = \frac{0.25 \text{ g} \times 1000 \text{ mg} \times 2 \text{ mL}}{400 \text{ mg} \quad 1 \text{ g}} = \underline{} \text{ mL}$$

6. Ordered: Cytarabine 350 mg IM daily
   Reconstitute with 3.5 mL of sterile water = 500 mg / mL

   $$X = \frac{350 \text{ mg}}{500 \text{ mg}} \times 1 \text{ mL} = 0.7 \text{ mL}$$

7. Ordered: Claforan (cetoxime) 665 mg IV BID
   Reconstitute 10 mL bacteriostatic water = 95 mg / mL

   $$X = \frac{665 \text{ mg}}{95 \text{ mg}} \times \text{mL} = 7 \text{ mL}$$

8. Methocarbamol 0.5 g IM QID
   Reconstitute with 20 mL sterile water = 1000 mg / 3 mL

   1 g = 1000 mg

   $$X = \frac{0.5 \text{ g} \times 1000 \text{ mg} \times 3 \text{ mL}}{1000 \text{ mg} \quad 1 \text{ g}} = 1.5 \text{ mL}$$

Answer Sheet

(Reconstituted Meds)

1) 10.5 mL / 2.1 teaspoon

2) 9 mL

3) 1.1 mL

4) 2.7 mL

5) 1.3 mL

6) 0.7 mL

7) 7 mL

8) 1.5 mL

General Reference

- The common cardiovascular medications are intended to provide some general information.

- It is not a complete discussion of these medications but guidelines and examples.

- Any questions or concerns, please discuss with qualified personnel or facility's protocols.

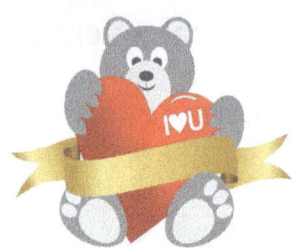

Cardiac Information

1. Ace Inhibitors (angiotensin-converting enzyme inhibitors)
   — Decrease blood pressure and fluid retention used for high blood pressure, heart failure, after a heart attack, and kidney protection in diabetic patients

2. Antiplatelet
   — Meds help to prevent blood clots from forming by keeping platelets in the body from sticking together
   — Also used to prevent heart attacks, strokes, and other medical problems

3. Beta Blockers
   — Are used to decrease blood pressure and heart rate
   — Other uses are to treat high blood pressure, angina, irregular heartbeats, heart failure, and after a heart attack to prevent further damage

4. Calcium Channel Blockers
   — Decrease blood pressure, some meds in this group help reduce heart rate and prevent heart vessel spasms
   — Used for high blood pressure, to prevent chest pain, irregular heart rhythms, coronary artery spasms

5. Digoxin
   — Helps the heart work better and control the heart rate
   — Used for heart failure and irregular heart rhythms

6. Diuretics
   — Reduce swelling and fluid retention caused by certain medical problems
   — Cause the kidneys to get rid of unneeded salt and water from the body into the urine
   — Used for high blood pressure and heart failure

7. Nitrates
   — Used to prevent chest pain (angina) or stop an attack of angina and dilates the blood vessels which decreases the workload on the heart

8. Potassium
   — Used to replace potassium from the body and prevent potassium deficiency than can be caused by certain disease or drugs

9. Receptor Activation Agonist:
   — Alpha 1: affects arteries, increases vascular tone, increase blood pressure and constriction
   — Alpha 2: dilatation
   — Beta 1: heart stimulation, increase heart rate, increase contractility increase arrhythmia, and increase cardiac output
   — Beta 2: bronchodilators, affect blood vessels, and **vasodilation**

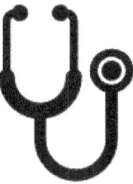

CO (cardiac output / cardiac index). The amount of blood that the heart pumps each minute, which measures the heart's ability to meet the body's oxygen demands. Body size does affect the overall cardiac output. The cardiac index is a more precise measurement of heart function.

Normal resting range is 4-8 L / min, including the body size.
Normal cardiac index is 2.6 – 4.2 L / min / m²

CO = SV x HR
CI = CO / BSA

One of the common causes of low cardiac output is low blood pressure. Other reasons include heart damage, abnormal heartbeats, or certain medications. This can be a cause of kidney failure and / or failure to other major organs.

- **Preload = volume of blood received by the heart.**
- Basically, **preload** is <u>stretch</u>.
- **Afterload = pressure or resistance the heart has to overcome to eject blood.**
- **Afterload** is <u>squeeze</u>.

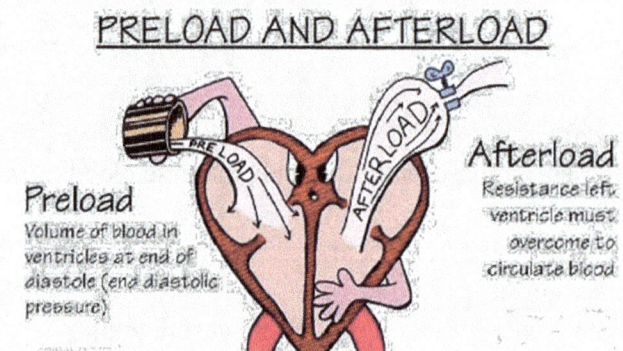

Preload

This occurs during diastoles with pulmonary blood filling the atria and stretching of the myocardial fibers. Preload is the filling pressure of the heart at the end of diastole.

The left atrial pressure (LAP) at the end of diastole will determine the preload. The greater the preload, the greater the volume of blood in the heart will be at the end of diastole.

Afterload

A resistance of the heart to successfully send blood into the aorta during every beat.

CVP (central venous pressure) A measure of blood volume and venous return. Its primary goal is to monitor fluid volume status. The CVP reflects right-sided ventricular end diastolic filling pressures (RVEDP). CVP is the clinical indicator of RV preload.

Normal range is 2–8 cm H²O or 2–6 mmHg

A decreased CVP may be caused by hypovolemia or decreased venous return and shock. The correction would be to initiate fluids to increase preload.

An increased CVP may be caused by fluid overload, increased venous return or right-sided cardiac failure, vasoconstriction, and cardiac tamponade. The improvement will be to a diuretic vasodilator to reduce after- load and treatment for cardiac tamponade.

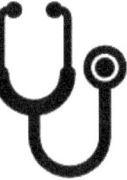

MAP (mean arterial pressure): The amount of arterial, which maintains adequate perfusion of all vital organs, usually 60 mmHg.

MAP = Systolic BP + 2 (Diastolic BP) / 3.

Normal 70-100 mmHg

Example: 128 + 2 (78) / 3 = ▓▓ MAP

Low MAP are possible signs of sepsis, stroke, and internal bleeding.

High MAP may indicate heart attack, kidney, and heart failure.

SVR (systemic vascular resistance):

The measurement of resistance of the systemic vascular bed to blood flow.

SVR is calculated by: SVR = (MAP–CVP) x 80 / cardiac output.

- A decreased SVR can be caused by early septic shock, vasodilators, morphine, nitrates, or hypercarbia.
- An increased SVR can be caused by vasoconstrictors, hypovolemia, or late septic shock.

PVR (pulmonary vascular resistance): The impediment of the pulmonary vascular bed to blood flow.

- A decreased PVR is caused by medications such as calcium channel blockers, aminophylline, or isoproterenol or by the delivery of O_2.
- An increased PVR or "Pulmonary Hypertension" is caused by pulmonary vascular disease, pulmonary embolism, or pulmonary vasculitis, or hypoxia.

SVI (stroke volume index): The amount of blood ejected from the heart in one cardiac cycle, relative to body surface area (BSA).

- A decreased SVI may be caused by CHF, late septic shock, beta-blockers, or an MI.
- An increased SVI can be indicative of early septic shock, hyperthermia, hypervolemia, or by medications.

PAWP (pulmonary artery wedge pressure):

It is used to assess left ventricular function (left ventricular end diastolic pressure).

The normal PAWP range is 8–12 mmHg.

- A high PAWP may indicate left ventricle failure, mitral valve pathology, cardiac insufficiency, cardiac compression post hemorrhage, and cardiac tamponade
- A low PAWP reflects hypovolemia.
- PWP is the clinical indicator of LV preload

Listed below are some medications that are detrimental to the cardiac system.

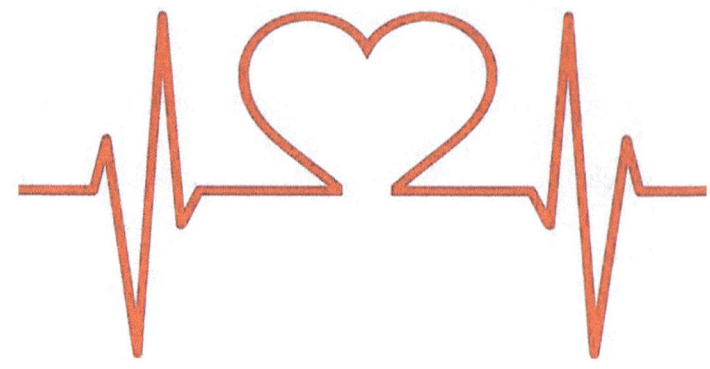

I. Drugs that afterload, SVR, PVR are arterial dilators:

- Alpha (Regitine)
- Amrinone
- Ca+ channel blockers
- Nitroglycerin
- Nitroprusside

II. Drugs that afterload, SVR, PVR are vasopressors:

- Dopamine
- Epinephrine
- Neosynephrine
- Norepinephrine

EXCELLENCE in NURSING MATH REVIEW

III. Drugs to contractility, SVI are beta-blockers:

- Atenolol
- Ca+ channel blockers
- Esmolol
- Labetolol
- Propranolol

IV. Drugs to contractility, SVI are positive inotropes:

- Digoxin
- Dopamine
- Dobutamine
- Milrinone

V. Drugs to preload, CVP, PAWP are venous dilators:

- Alpha & Ca+ channel blockers
- Amrinone
- Nitroglycerin
- Nitroprusside
- Diuretics:
    - Bumex
    - Furosemide
    - Mannitol

VI. Drugs to preload, CVP, PAWP

- Volume
- Blood
- Colloid
- Crystalloids
- Hetastarch

Here are a few meds listed as vasopressors:

- Dobutamine
- Dopamine
- Epinephrine
- Milrinone
- Norepinephrine
- Phenylephrine
- Vasopressin

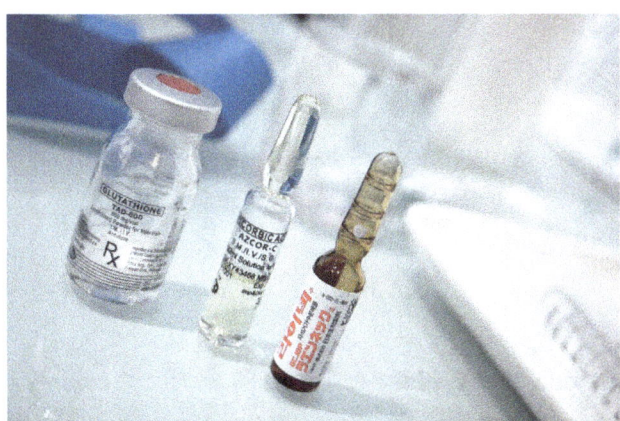

Guidelines for IV Critical Care Meds

- Dimensional analysis can be used to calculate the flow rate in mL / hr.

- The safest approach to drug calculations is to use the same method for the same type of problem each time.

- Intravenous therapy is the fastest way to deliver fluids and medications directly into a vein through- out the body.

- Some medications have a rapid action and / or short duration frequently titrated within specific dosage per flow rate to elicit a measurable physiologic response.

- Medication is titrated at the lowest dosage ordered and increased or decreased slowly to obtain the desired response.

- Generic (small letters) and brand names (capitalized letters) are used interchangeably.

- Always check daily weight before administering meds.

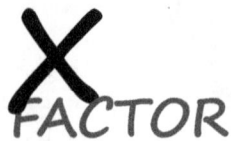

Calculating IV Meds

- This workbook includes the *x factor* formula.

  The *x factor* is the unknown variable.

  Always divide desired dose into *x factor*.

- All calculations are examples.

- The goal is to determine the correct rate to set the IV pump.

- Most diluents are D5W, normal saline, 1 / 2 normal saline, and lactated ringers.

- Some meds exhibit bolus or loading doses before maintenance doses.

For this workbook, round to the nearest thousandth place value to determine the *x factor*.

Round to the nearest tenth place value for mL per hour.

Rounding Rules

Example:

8.7245 = 9 Rounded to whole number

= 8.7 Rounded to one decimal place (10th)

= 8.72 Rounded to two decimal places (100th)

= 8.725 Rounded to three decimal places (1000th)

EXCELLENCE in NURSING MATH REVIEW

Guidelines of IV Calculations

Microgram per kilogram per minute (mcg / kg / min)

Microgram per minute (mcg / min)

Milligram per minute (mg / min)

Milligram per hour (mg / hr)

Note: Some medications are calculated based on mcg / kg / min

                                               mcg / min

                                               mg / kg / hr

kg interprets that most medications are weight based.

The following **tools** can be helpful in calculating mL / hr. (hourly rate).

1. $\dfrac{\text{Dose (mcg / kg / min) x wt (kg) x drug volume (mL) x 60 (min / hr)}}{\text{drug concentration in mcg}} = \text{mL / hr.}$

2. $\dfrac{\text{Dose (mcg / min) x drug volume in mL x 60 (min / hr)}}{\text{drug concentration in mcg}} = \text{mL / hr.}$

3. $\dfrac{\text{Dose (mg / kg / hr) x wt (kg) x drug volume (mL)}}{\text{drug concentration (mg)}} = \text{mL / hr.}$

Reminders:

- If the dosage calculation is in mg / min or mcg / min, **add 60 minutes** into the formula.

- If the dosage calculation is in mg / hr. or mg / kg / hr., **remove 60 minutes** from the formula.

- If the dosage calculation does not require weight, **remove wt.** from the formula.

Tool #4:

$$\text{Time} = \frac{\text{volume}}{\text{time}} = \text{flow rate with fractional hours}$$

Tool #5

$$\frac{\text{mcg} \times \text{kg} \times \text{min}}{\text{drug concentration}} = \text{mL/hr}$$

Drug Concentration (premixed solution) = mg / mL = mg x 1000 mcg / mL

Example: 400 mg / 250 mL = 1.6 mg x 1000 mcg = 1600 mcg / mL

Hint:

The *x factor* remains unchanged in the same equation unless there is a change in the premixed solutions (drug concentrations) or weight in kilograms.

Again, 1 mg = 1000 mcg

Let's

Work

Together

EXCELLENCE in NURSING MATH REVIEW

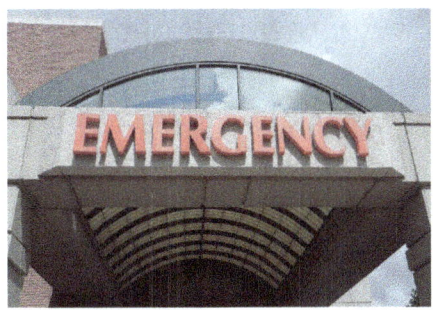

MCG / KG / MIN

Acova (argatroban)

Anticoagulant is used to prevent blood clots in clients with low platelets (thrombocytopenia) due to heparin (HIT) injury.

Range: 0.3 to 25 mcg / kg / min

Drug concentrations: 250 mg / 250 mg   500 mL / 500 mL

Pt's weight: 84 kg

Physician ordered: 2 mcg / kg / min

1. Calculate *x factor* = $\dfrac{250 \text{ mg} \times (1000 \text{ mcg}) / 84 \text{kg} / 60 \text{ min}}{250 \text{ mL}}$ = ____ *xf*

2. Determine mL / hr. = $\dfrac{2 \text{ mcg / kg / min (ordered)}}{xf \,(x\,factor)}$ = ____ mL / hr.

3. Double check for accuracy = rate on pump x *(x factor)* = mcg / kg / min

   ____ mL / hr. x ____ *xf* = ____ mcg / kg / min

Aggrastat (tirofiban)

An anti-platelet drug indicated to reduce the rate of thrombotic cardiovascular events and used in treatment of non-ST elevation acute coronary syndrome.

Drug concentrations: $\underline{5 \text{ mg}}$ $\underline{12.5 \text{ mg}}$ $\underline{25 \text{mg}}$
                    100 mL   250 mL   500 mL

Range: 25 mcg / kg BOLUS (most patients)

    0.15 mcg / kg / min if CrCl > 60 mL / min

    0.075 mcg / kg / min if CrCl < 60 mL / min

Pt's weight: 86 lbs. = ▓ kg

Physician ordered: 0.15 mcg / kg / min

1. Calculate $x\ factor$ = $\underline{5 \text{ mg}}$ x (▓ mcg) / ▓ kg / 60 min = ▓ xf
                    100 mL

2. Determine mL / hr = $\dfrac{\text{▓ mcg / kg / min (ordered)}}{\text{▓ xf } (x\ factor)}$ = ▓ mL / hr

3. Double check for accuracy = rate on pump x ($x\ factor$) = mcg / kg / min

    ▓ mL / hr x ▓ xf = ▓ mcg / kg / min

Brevibloc (esmolol)

An antiarrhythmic and beta-blocker used to reduce heart rate, blood pressure, and improve contractility.

Range: 25 to 300 mcg / kg / min

Drug concentrations: $\underline{2000 \text{ mg}} \quad \underline{2500 \text{ mg}}$
$100 \text{ mL} \quad 250 \text{ mL}$

Pt's weight: 65 kg

Physician ordered: 50 mcg / kg / min

1. Calculate $x\ factor = \dfrac{2500 \text{ mg} \times (1{,}000 \text{ mcg})}{250 \text{ mL}} / 65 \text{ kg} /\ \_\_\_ \text{ min} = \_\_\_ xf$

2. Determine mL / hr. = $\dfrac{\_\_\_ \text{ mcg / kg / min (ordered)}}{\_\_\_ \ xf\ (x\ factor)} = \_\_\_$ mL / hr

3. Double check for accuracy = rate on pump x (x factor) = mcg / kg / min

   ___ mL / hr x ___ xf = ___ mcg / kg / min

Corlopam (fenoldopam)

This medication is a vasodilator, which is used for severe malignant and hypertensive emergencies.

Drug concentrations: $\dfrac{10 \text{ mg}}{250 \text{ mL}}$ $\dfrac{20 \text{ mg}}{500 \text{ mL}}$ $\dfrac{40 \text{ mg}}{1000 \text{ mL}}$

Range: 0.03 to 1.6 mcg / kg / min

Weight: ▓ kg (154 lbs.)

Physician ordered: 0.05 mcg / kg / min

1. Calculate concentration = $\dfrac{10 \text{ mg} \times (1000 \text{ mcg})}{250 \text{ mL}}$ = ▓ mcg / mL

2. Determine *x factor*: $\dfrac{40 \text{ mcg} / 70 \text{kg} / 60 \text{ min}}{\text{mL}}$ = ▓ *xf*

3. Determine mL / hr. = $\dfrac{\text{▓ mcg x ▓ kg x ▓ min (ordered)}}{\text{▓ concentration (mcg / mL)}}$ = ▓ mL / hr

4. Double check for accuracy: rate on pump x *(x factor)* = mcg / kg / min

   ▓ mL / hr x ▓ *xf* = ▓ mcg / kg / min

Diprivan (propofol)

This medication is a short-term sedation, which includes monitoring serum triglyceride levels, reducing blood pressure, and / or cardiac output.

Range: 5 to 100 mcg / kg / min

Drug concentrations: 500 mg / 50 mL   1000 mg / 100 mL   500 mg / 250 mL

Pt's weight: 220 lbs = (___ kg)

Physician ordered: 5 mcg / kg / min

1. Calculate x factor = $\dfrac{500 \text{ mg}}{50 \text{ mL}}$ x (___ mcg) / 100 kg / ___ min = ___ xf

2. Determine mL / hr = $\dfrac{\text{___ mcg / kg / min (ordered)}}{\text{___ xf (x factor)}}$ = ___ mL / hr

3. Double check for accuracy = rate on pump x (x factor) = mcg / kg / min

    ___ mL / hr x ___ xf = ___ mcg / kg / min

Example #2: propofol

Physician ordered: 40 mcg / kg / min

Drug concentration: 1000 mg / 100 mL

Pt's weight: 138 lbs (____ kg)

1. Calculate *x factor* = $\frac{\text{1000 mg}}{\text{100 mL}}$ x (1,000 mcg) / ____ kg / 60 min = ____ *xf*

2. Determine mL / hr = 40 $\frac{\text{mcg / kg / min (ordered)}}{\text{____ } \textit{xf} \text{ (x factor)}}$ = ____ mL / hr

3. Double check for accuracy = rate on pump x (*x factor*) = mcg / kg / min

   ____ mL / hr x ____ *xf* = ____ mcg / kg / min

EXCELLENCE in NURSING MATH REVIEW

Example #3: propofol

IV pump set @ 35 mL / hr

Drug concentration: 500 mg / 250 mL

Pt's weight: 115 lbs = (____ kg)

1. Calculate *x factor* = $\dfrac{500 \text{ mg}}{250 \text{ mL}}$ × (1,000 mcg) / ____ kg / 60 min = ____ *xf*

2. Determine mcg / kg / min = 35 mL / hr × ____ *(x factor)* = ____ mcg / kg / min

3. Double check for accuracy = ____ $\dfrac{\text{mcg / kg / min}}{\text{____ } xf \text{ (x factor)}}$ = ____ mL / hr

practice

practice

practice

practice

Dobutrex (dobutamine hydrochloride)

An adrenergic medication that is used to increase cardiac output.

Range: 2 to 40 mcg / kg / min

Drug concentrations: $\dfrac{250 \text{ mg}}{250 \text{ mL}}$ $\dfrac{500 \text{ mg}}{250 \text{ mL}}$ $\dfrac{1250 \text{ mg}}{250 \text{ mL}}$

Pt's weight: 85 kg

Physician ordered: 10 mcg / kg / min

Example:

1. Calculate *x factor* = $\dfrac{250 \text{ mg}}{250 \text{ mL}}$ x (1,000 mcg) / 85 kg / 60 min = 0.196 *xf*

2. Determine mL / hr = $\dfrac{10 \text{ mcg / kg / min (ordered)}}{0.196 \text{ xf (x factor)}}$ = 51 mL / hr

3. Double check for *accuracy* = rate on pump x *(x factor)* = mcg / kg / min

    51 mL / hr x 0.196 *xf* = 9.9 mcg / kg / min

Dopamine

An adrenergic and vasopressor drug used to correct hypotension.

Range: 1 to 50 mcg / kg / min

Drug concentrations: $\dfrac{400 \text{ mg}}{250 \text{ mL}}$ $\dfrac{800 \text{ mg}}{250 \text{ mL}}$ $\dfrac{800 \text{ mg}}{500 \text{ mL}}$

Pt's weight: 70 kg

Physician ordered: 5 mcg / kg / min

1. Calculate *x factor* = $\dfrac{400 \text{ mg}}{250 \text{ mL}}$ x (▒ mcg) / ▒ kg / 60 min = ▒ *xf*

2. Determine mL / hr = $\dfrac{\text{▒ mcg / kg / min (ordered)}}{\text{▒ } xf \text{ (x factor)}}$ = ▒ mL / hr

3. Double check for accuracy = rate on pump x (*x factor*) = mcg / kg / min

   ▒ mL / hr x ▒ *xf* = ▒ mcg / kg / min

Example #2: dopamine

Drug concentration: 800 mg / 500 mL or (1600 mcg / mL)

Pt's weight: 250 lbs = (▓ kg)

Physician ordered: 15 mcg / kg / min

1. Calculate *x factor* = 800 mg x (▓ mcg) / 113.6 kg / ▓ min = ▓ *xf*
   500 mL

2. Determine mL / hr = ▓ mcg / kg / min (ordered) = ▓ mL / hr
                        ▓ *xf* (*x factor*)

3. Double check for accuracy = rate on pump x (*x factor*) = mcg / kg / min

   ▓ mL / hr x ▓ *xf* = ▓ mcg / kg / min

EXCELLENCE in NURSING MATH REVIEW

Inocor (inamrinone lactate)

This medication produces vasodilation and treats short-term management of congestive heart failure (CHF).

Range: 2.5 to 15 mcg / kg / min

Drug concentrations: 300 mg   300 mg   500 mg
                      120 mL   300 mL   250 mL

Pt's weight: 137.6 lbs = (____ kg)

Physician ordered: 3.5 mcg / kg / min

1. Calculate *x factor* = $\frac{300 \text{ mg}}{120 \text{ mL}}$ x (____ mcg) / 62.5 kg / ____ min = ____ *xf*

2. Determine mL / hr = $\frac{\underline{ \text{mcg / kg / min (ordered)}}}{ \textit{xf} \, (x \, factor)}$ = ____ mL / hr

3. Double check for accuracy = rate on pump x (*x factor*) = mcg / kg / min

   ____ mL / hr x ____ *xf* = ____ mcg / kg / min

Integrilin (eptifibatide)

This medication is used to treat unstable angina, acute coronary syndrome, and non-Q-wave myocardial infarction.

Range: 0.5 to 2 mcg / kg / min

Drug concentrations: $\dfrac{75 \text{ mg}}{100 \text{ mL}}$ $\dfrac{200 \text{ mg}}{100 \text{ mL}}$

Pt's weight: 110 kg

Physician ordered: 1.5 mcg / kg / min

1. Calculate *x factor* = $\dfrac{75 \text{ mg}}{100 \text{ mL}}$ x (▮ mcg) / ▮ kg / ▮ min = ▮ xf

2. Determine mL / hr = $\dfrac{▮ \text{ mcg / kg / min (ordered)}}{▮ \text{ } xf \text{ } (x\text{ }factor)}$ = ▮ mL / hr

3. Double check for accuracy = rate on pump x (*x factor*) = mcg / kg / min

   ▮ mL / hr x ▮ *xf* = ▮ mcg / kg / min

Natrecor (nesiritide)

A vasodilator used in the management of CHF.

Range: 0.01 to 0.03 mcg / kg / min

Drug concentration: $\dfrac{1.5 \text{ mg}}{250 \text{ mL}}$

Pt's weight: 176 lbs = (▓ kg)

Physician ordered: 0.01 mcg / kg / min

1. Calculate *x factor*: $\dfrac{1.5 \text{ mg}}{250 \text{ mL}}$ x 1,000 mcg / 80 kg / 60 min = ▓ xf

2. Determine mL / hr = $\dfrac{\text{▓ mcg / kg / min (ordered)}}{\text{▓ xf (x factor)}}$ = ▓ mL / hr

3. Double check for accuracy: rate on pump x *(x factor)* = ▓ mcg / kg / min

   ▓ mL / hr x 0.001 *xf* = ▓ mcg / kg / min

Nimbex (cisatracurium besylate)

This medication is a neuromuscular blockade (paralytic) used to facilitate tracheal intubations and provide skeletal muscle relaxation.

Range: 0.5 to 10.2 mcg / kg / min

Drug concentrations: $\dfrac{100 \text{ mg}}{50 \text{ mL}}$ $\dfrac{100 \text{ mg}}{250 \text{ mL}}$

Pt's weight: 79 kg

Physician ordered: 6.5 mcg / kg / min

1. Calculate *x factor* = $\dfrac{100 \text{ mg}}{50 \text{ mL}}$ x (___ mcg) / ___ kg / 60 min = ___ *xf*

2. Determine mL / hr = $\dfrac{\text{___ mcg / kg / min (ordered)}}{\text{___ } xf\,(x\,factor)}$ = ___ mL / hr

3. Double check for accuracy = rate on pump x (*x factor*) = mcg / kg / min

    ___ mL / hr x ___ *xf* = ___ mcg / kg / min

EXCELLENCE in NURSING MATH REVIEW

Nipride (nitroprusside sodium)

A vasodilator, which is used to reduce blood pressure during a hypertensive crisis.

Range: 0.25 to 8 mcg / kg / min

Drug concentrations: $\frac{50 \text{ mg}}{250 \text{ mL}}$ $\frac{100 \text{ mg}}{250 \text{ mL}}$ $\frac{250 \text{ mg}}{250 \text{ mL}}$

Pt's weight: 132 lbs = (▓ kg)

Physician ordered: 3 mcg / kg / min

1. Calculate *x factor* = $\frac{100 \text{ mg} \times 1000 \text{ mcg} / \text{▓ kg} / \text{▓ min}}{250 \text{ mL}}$ = ▓ *xf*

2. Determine mL / hr = $\frac{\text{▓ mcg / kg / min (ordered)}}{\text{▓ } xf \text{ (x factor)}}$ = ▓ mL / hr

3. Double check for accuracy = rate on pump x (*x factor*) = mcg / kg / min

   ▓ mL / hr x ▓ *xf* = ▓ mcg / kg / min

Norcuron (vecuronium bromide)

Neuromuscular blocking medication is used to induce skeletal muscle relaxation during surgery or promote mechanical ventilation, and during pregnancy when benefits over-ride potential risks.

Range: 0.8 to 2 mcg / kg / min

Drug concentrations: 20 mg / 100 mL   50 mg / 50 mL   100 mg / 100 mL

Pt's weight: 78 kg

Physician ordered: 1.3 mcg / kg / min

1. Calculate x *factor* = $\frac{50 \text{ mg}}{50 \text{ mL}}$ x (▩ mcg) / (▩ kg) / ▩ min = ▩ *xf*

2. Determine mL / hr = $\frac{\text{▩ mcg / kg / min (ordered)}}{\text{▩ } xf \,(x\,factor)}$ = ▩ mL / hr

3. Double check for accuracy = rate on pump x (*x factor*) = mcg / kg / min

    ▩ mL / hr x ▩ *xf* = ▩ mcg / kg / min

EXCELLENCE in NURSING MATH REVIEW

Pavulon (pancuronium bromide)

A non-depolarizing neuromuscular blockade medication used to promote mechanical ventilation, intubation, and oxygen consumption. May reduce respiratory rate.

Drug concentrations: $\dfrac{50 \text{ mg}}{100 \text{ mL}}$ $\dfrac{100 \text{ mg}}{100 \text{ mL}}$ $\dfrac{12.5 \text{ mg}}{250 \text{ mL}}$

Range: 1 to 1.7 mcg / kg / min

Physician ordered: 1.2 mcg / kg / min

Pt's weight: 104 kg (228.8 lbs)

1. Calculate x factor = $\dfrac{100 \text{ mg}}{100 \text{ mL}}$ x (1000 mcg) / 104 kg / 60 min = ▒ xf

2. Determine mL / hr = $\dfrac{\text{▒ mcg / kg / min (ordered)}}{\text{▒ xf (x factor)}}$ = ▒ mL / hr

3. Double check for accuracy = rate on pump x (x factor) = mcg / kg / min

    ▒ mL / hr x ▒ xf = ▒ mcg / kg / min

Primacor (milrinone lactate)

This medication is classified as a positive inotrope, which is used to produce vasodilatation and short-term treatment of CHF. This is useful for acute management of low cardiac output.

Range: 0.375 to 0.75 mcg / kg / min

Drug concentrations: $\dfrac{20\text{ mg}}{100\text{ mL}}$ $\dfrac{40\text{ mg}}{200\text{ mL}}$ $\dfrac{50\text{ mg}}{250\text{ mL}}$

Pt's weight: 158.4 lbs = (____ kg)

Physician ordered: 0.375 mcg / kg / min

1. Calculate *x factor* = $\dfrac{20\text{ mg}}{100\text{ mL}}$ x (____ mcg) / ____ kg / ____ min = ____ *xf*

2. Determine mL / hr = $\dfrac{\underline{\text{____ mcg / kg / min (ordered)}}}{\text{____ } xf \text{ (}x\text{ factor)}}$ = ____ mL / hr

3. Double check for accuracy = rate on pump x (*x factor*) = mcg / kg / min

   ____ mL / hr x ____ *xf* = ____ mcg / kg / min

EXCELLENCE in NURSING MATH REVIEW

Example #2: Primacor

Drug concentration: 40 mg / 200 mL

Pt's weight: 101 kg

Physician ordered: 0.495 mcg / kg / min

1. Calculate *x factor* = $\frac{40 \text{ mg}}{200 \text{ mL}}$ x (____ mcg) / ____ kg / 60 min = ____ *xf*

2. Determine mL / hr = $\frac{\text{____ mcg / kg / min (ordered)}}{\text{____ xf (x factor)}}$ = ____ mL / hr

3. Double check for accuracy = rate on pump x (*x factor*) = mcg / kg / min

    ____ mL / hr x ____ *xf* = ____ mcg / kg / min

practice

practice

practice

practice

Example #3: Primacor

Drug concentration: 50 mg / 250 mL

Pt's weight: 159 lbs = (▓ kg)

Physician ordered: 0.75 mcg / kg / min

1. Calculate *x factor* = $\underline{50\ mg}$ x (1000 mcg) / ▓ kg / ▓ min = ▓ *xf*
   250 mL

2. Determine mL / hr = $\dfrac{\text{▓ mcg / kg / min (ordered)}}{\text{▓ } xf\ (x\ factor)}$ = ▓ mL / hr

3. Double check for accuracy = rate on pump x (*x factor*) = mcg / kg / min

   ▓ mL / hr x ▓ *xf* = ▓ mcg / kg / min

Zemuron (rocuronium)

Drug concentration: 50 mg / 50 mL

Range: 4 to 16 mcg / kg / min

Pt's weight: 95 kg

Physician ordered: 12 mcg / kg / min

Example:

1. *x factor* = 50 mg x (1000 mcg) / 95 kg / 60 min / 50 mL = 0.175 *xf*

2. Ordered = $\dfrac{12 \text{ mcg / kg / min}}{0.175 xf}$ = 68.5 mL / hr

3. Double check for accuracy = 68.5 mL / hr x 0.175 *xf* = 12 mcg / kg / min

Answer Sheet

(Mcg / Kg / Min)

Drugs	X factor	mL / hr	Concentration
Argatroban	0.198	10.1	1,000 mcg / mL
Tirofiban	0.021	7	50 mcg / mL
Esmolol	2.564	19.5	10,000 mcg / mL
Fenoldopam	0.009	5.3	40 mcg / mL
Propofol #1	1.666	3.15	10,000 mcg / mL
#2	2.658	22.3	
#3	0.638		2,000 mcg / mL
Dobutamine	0.196	51	1,000 mcg / mL
Inotropin #1	0.38	13.1	1,600 mcg / mL
#2	0.234	63.9	
Inamrinone	0.666	5.3	2,500 mcg / mL
Eptifibatide	0.113	13.2	750 mcg / mL
Nesiritide	0.001	10	6 mcg / mL
Cisatracurium	0.421	15.4	2,000 mcg / mL
Nitroprusside	0.111	27	400 mcg / mL
Vecuronium	0.213	6.1	1,000 mcg / mL
Pancuronium	0.16	7.5	1,000 mcg / mL
Milrinone #1	0.046	8.1	200 mcg / mL
#2	0.033	15	
#3	0.046	16.3	
Rocuronium	0.175	68.4	1,000 mcg / mL

Mcg / Min

Adrenaline (epinephrine)

This medication is used for bronchospasm, anaphylaxis reaction, and to restore rhythm in a cardiac arrest. The category is vasopressor / cardiac stimulant—an alpha 1 and beta 1 agonist.

Range: 1 to 5 mcg / min

Drug concentrations: $\dfrac{1\text{ mg}}{250\text{ mL}}$ $\dfrac{5\text{ mg}}{250\text{ mL}}$ $\dfrac{10\text{ mg}}{50\text{ mL}}$

Physician ordered: 3 mcg / min

1. Calculate $x\ factor = \dfrac{5\text{mg}}{250\text{ mL}} \times (1{,}000\text{ mcg}) / 60\text{ min} = 0.333xf$

2. Determine mL / hr = $\dfrac{3\text{ mcg / min (ordered)}}{0.333xf\ (x\ factor)} = 9\text{ mL / hr}$

3. Double check for accuracy = rate on pump x (*x factor*) = mcg / min

    9 mL / hr x 0.333 *xf* = 3 mcg / min

Isuprel (isoproterenol hydrochloride)

The medication is used to treat bronchial asthma and reverses bronchospasm.

Isuprel is in the beta agonist classification.

Range: 2 to 30 mcg / min

Drug concentrations: $\dfrac{1 \text{ mg}}{250 \text{ mL}}$ $\dfrac{2 \text{ mg}}{500 \text{ mL}}$

Physician ordered: 4 mcg / min

1. Calculate $x\,factor = \dfrac{2 \text{ mg}}{500 \text{ mL}} \times (\_\_ \text{ mcg}) / \_\_ \text{ min} = \_\_ xf$

2. Determine mL / hr = $\dfrac{\_\_ \text{ mcg / min (ordered)}}{\_\_ xf\,(x\,factor)}$ = __ mL / hr

3. Double check = rate on pump x ($x\,factor$) = mcg / min

   __ mL / hr x __ xf = __ mcg / min

EXCELLENCE in NURSING MATH REVIEW

Levophed (norepinephrine)

This medication is considered a vasopressor and used to restore blood pressure during hypotensive crisis—an alpha 1 and 2 agonist.

Range: 0.5 to 30 mcg / min

Drug concentrations: $\dfrac{4 \text{ mg}}{250 \text{ mL}}$ $\dfrac{8 \text{ mg}}{250 \text{ mL}}$ $\dfrac{16 \text{ mg}}{250 \text{ mL}}$

Physician ordered: 15 mcg / min

Initially 8 to 12 mcg / min (bolus) then maintenance dose

1. Calculate *x factor* = $\dfrac{16 \text{ mg}}{250 \text{ mL}}$ x (____ mcg) / ____ min = ____ *xf*

2. Determine mL / hr = $\dfrac{\_\_\_\_ \text{ mcg / min (ordered)}}{\_\_\_\_ \text{ xf (x factor)}}$ = ____ mL / hr

3. Double check = rate on pump x *(x factor)* = mcg / min

    ____ mL / hr x ____ *xf* = ____ mcg / min

Example #2: Levophed

Premixed solution: 4 mg / 250 mL

Physician ordered: 10 mcg / min

1. Calculate *x factor* : 4 mg x 1000 mcg / 60 min / 250 mL = ▒ *xf*

2. Determine mL / hr = $\dfrac{10 \text{ mcg / min (ordered)}}{\text{▒ } xf \text{ (x factor)}}$ = ▒ mL / hr

3. Double check = rate on pump x (*x factor*) = mcg / min

    ▒ mL / hr x ▒ *xf* = ▒ mcg / min

Neosynephrine (phenylephrine)

The goal is to treat mild to moderate hypotensive emergencies during a cardiac crisis.

Range: 10 to 220 mcg / min

Drug concentrations: $\frac{10 \text{ mg}}{250 \text{ mL}}$ $\frac{40 \text{ mg}}{250 \text{ mL}}$ $\frac{80 \text{ mg}}{250 \text{ mL}}$

Physician ordered: 20 mcg / min

1. Calculate *x factor*: $\frac{10 \text{ mg}}{250 \text{ mL}}$ x (___ mcg) / ___ min = ___ *xf*

2. Determine mL / hr = $\frac{\_\_\_ \text{ mcg / min (ordered)}}{\_\_\_ \text{ xf (x factor)}}$ = ___ mL / hr

3. Double check = rate on pump x (*x factor*) = mcg / min

   ___ mL / hr x ___ *xf* = ___ mcg / min

Tridil (nitroglycerin)

A nitrate that treats congestive heart failure, hypertension, chest pain, and myocardial infarction.

Range: 1 to 300 mcg / min

Drug concentrations: 25 mg / 250 mL   50 mg / 250 mL   100 mg / 250 mL

Physician ordered: 50 mcg / min

1. Calculate $x\,factor = \dfrac{25\,mg \times (\underline{\quad}\,mcg)\,/\,\underline{\quad}\,min}{250\,mL} = \underline{\quad}\,xf$

2. Determine $mL/hr = \dfrac{\underline{\quad}\,mcg/min\,(ordered)}{\underline{\quad}\,xf\,(x\,factor)} = \underline{\quad}\,mL/hr$

3. Double check = rate on pump x (x factor) = mcg / min

   $\underline{\quad}\,mL/hr \times \underline{\quad}\,xf = \underline{\quad}\,mcg/min$

EXCELLENCE in NURSING MATH REVIEW

Example #2: Tridil

1. Physician ordered = ▓ mcg / min

2. Premixed solution: 50 mg / 250 mL

3. **IV Pump = 5 mL / hr**

   $$X = \frac{5 \text{ mL}}{\text{hr}} \times \frac{1 \text{ hr}}{60 \text{ min}} \times \frac{50 \text{ mg}}{250 \text{ mL}} \times \frac{1{,}000 \text{ mcg}}{1 \text{ mg}} = \frac{250000}{15000} = 16.6 \text{ mcg / min}$$

   Double check = *x factor* = (50 mg x 1,000 mcg / 60 min / 250 mL) = 3.333*xf*

   $$\frac{16.6 \text{ mcg / min}}{3.333 \text{ xf}} = 5 \text{ mL / hr}$$

Answer Sheet

(Mcg / Min)

Drugs	X factor	mL / hr	Concentration (mcg / mL)
Epinephrine	0.333	9	20
Isoproterenol	0.066	60	4
Norepinephrine #1	1.066	14.1	64
#2	0.266	37.5	16
Phenylephrine	0.666	30	40
Nitroglycerin #1	1.666	30	100
#2	3.333	5	200

EXCELLENCE in NURSING MATH REVIEW

LET'S PRACTICE

Mg / Min

Converting mg / min. You are doing great.

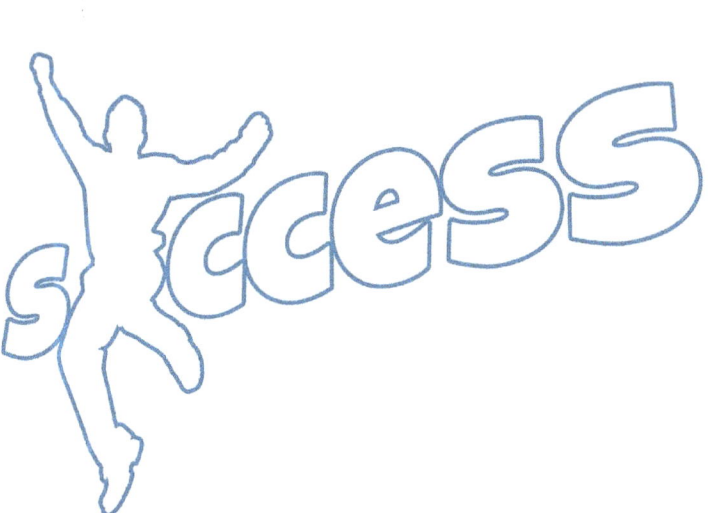

Cordarone (amiodarone hydrochloride)

This medication is used to treat stable wide complex tachycardia arrhythmias.

Range: 0.5 to 1 mg / min

Premixed solutions:

150 mg	900 mg	450 mg	900 mg
100 mL	150 mL	250 mL	500 mL

Ordered: 0.5 mg / min

Example:

- Determine $x\ factor$ = 450 mg / 60 min / 250 mL = 0.03 xf

- Determine mL / hr = $\dfrac{0.5\ mg\ /\ min\ (ordered)}{0.03\ (x\ factor)}$ = 16.7 mL / hr

- Double check = rate on pump x ($x\ factor$) = mg / min

    16.7 mL / hr x 0.03xf = 0.5 mg / min

- Reconfirm: $\dfrac{0.5\ mg}{min} \times \dfrac{60\ min}{hr} \times \dfrac{250\ mL}{450\ mg}$ = ▩ mL / hr

EXCELLENCE in NURSING MATH REVIEW

Trandate (labetolol)

A beta-blocker used for the treatment of hypertension.

Range: 0.5 to 5 mg / min

Premixed solutions:
200 mg	300 mg	480 mg
160 mL	240 mL	600 mL

Ordered: 2 mg / min

- Determine drug concentration: 300 mg / 240 mL (___ mg / mL)

- Determine mL / hr = $\dfrac{\text{___ mg / min (ordered)} \times 60 \text{ min}}{\text{___ (drug concentration)}}$ = ___ mL / hr

- Double check = $\dfrac{2 \text{ mg}}{\text{min}} \times \dfrac{240 \text{ mL}}{300 \text{ mg}} \times \dfrac{60 \text{ min}}{\text{hr}}$ = ___ mL / hr

Xylocaine (lidocaine hydrochloride)

This medication is used in the treatment of ventricular arrhythmias.

Range: 1 to 4 mg / min

Premixed solutions: $\underline{1 g}$ $\underline{2 g}$ $\underline{2 g}$
 125 mL   250 mL   500 mL

*Remember 1g = 1000 mg

Ordered: 3 mg / min

- Determine *x factor* = 1 g x 1000 mg / 60 min / 125 mL = ▒ *xf*

- Determine mL / hr = ▒ mg / min (ordered) = ▒ mL / hr
  ▒ *xf* (*x factor*)

- Double check = rate on pump x (*x factor*) = mg / min

  ▒ mL / hr x ▒ *xf* = ▒ mg / min

- Reconfirm: 3 mg x 125 mL x 60 min = ▒ mL / hr
  min   1000 mg   hr

EXCELLENCE in NURSING MATH REVIEW

Example #2: Xylocaine

Drug concentration: 2 g / 250 mL

Ordered: 4 mg / min

$$X = \frac{4 \text{ mg}}{\text{min}} \times \frac{60 \text{ min}}{1 \text{ hr}} \times \frac{1 \text{ g}}{1000 \text{ mg}} \times \frac{250 \text{ mL}}{2 \text{ g}} = \underline{\quad} \text{ mL / hr}$$

- Double check = 2g x 1000 mg / 60 min / 250 mL = ___ xf

$$\textbf{Ordered} = \frac{4 \text{ mg / min}}{0.133xf} = \underline{\quad} \text{ mL / hr}$$

- Reconfirm: ___ mL / hr x ___ xf (x factor) = ___ mg / min

Epsom Salt (magnesium sulfate)

This medication is used in torsade's de pointe, hypo-magnesium, adjunct for ventricular tachycardia, and ventricular fibrillation.

Range: 3 to 20 mg / min

Premixed solution: 4g / 100 mL

Ordered: 3 mg / min

- Determine *x factor* = $\dfrac{4\,g \times (\underline{\quad} mg)}{100\,mL} / \underline{\quad} min = \underline{\quad} xf$

- Determine mL / hr = $\dfrac{\underline{\quad}\, mg/min\,(ordered)}{\underline{\quad}\, xf\,(x\,factor)} = \underline{\quad} mL/hr$

- Double check = rate on pump x *(x factor)* = mg / min

    $\underline{\quad}$ mL / hr x $\underline{\quad}$ *xf (x factor)* = $\underline{\quad}$ mg / min

- Reconfirm: $\dfrac{3\,mg}{min} \times \dfrac{100\,mL}{4000\,mg} \times \dfrac{60\,min}{hr} = \underline{\quad} mL/hr$

Example #2: magnesium sulfate

Ordered: 15 mg / min

Premixed solution: 4 g / 100 mL

$$X = \frac{15 \text{ mg}}{\text{min}} \times \frac{60 \text{ min}}{1 \text{ hr}} \times \frac{1 \text{ g}}{1000 \text{ mg}} \times \frac{100 \text{ mL}}{4 \text{ g}} = \underline{} \text{ mL / hr}$$

- Double check = 4g x 1000 mg / 60 min / 100 mL = ___ xf

- **Ordered:** ___ mg / min = ___ mL / hr
              ___ xf (x factor)

Pronestyl (procainamide hydrochloride)

The medication is used to prevent recurrent life-threatening ventricular arrhythmias.

Range: 1 to 50 mg / min

Premixed solutions: $\dfrac{2g}{250 \text{ mL}}$ $\dfrac{4g}{250 \text{ mL}}$

Ordered: 3 mg / min

- Determine x factor = 4 g x (▒ mg) / ▒ min / ▒ mL = ▒ xf

- Determine mL / hr = $\dfrac{\text{▒ ordered}}{\text{▒ } xf\,(x\,factor)}$ = ▒ mL / hr

- Double Check = rate on pump x ($x\,factor$) = mg / min

    ▒ mL / hr x ▒ xf = ▒ mg / min

- Reconfirm: $\dfrac{\text{▒ ordered x 60 min}}{\text{▒ drug concentration}}$ = ▒ mL / hr

Answer Sheet

(Mg / Min)

Drugs	X factor	mL / hr	Concentration (mg / mL)
Amiodarone	0.03	16.7	1.8
Labetolol	0.021	96	1.25
Lidocaine #1	0.133	22.5	8
#2	*	30	*
Magnesium Sulfate #1	0.666	4.5	40
#2	*	22.5	*
Procainamide	0.266	11.3	16

Now. try these practice problems…mg / hr

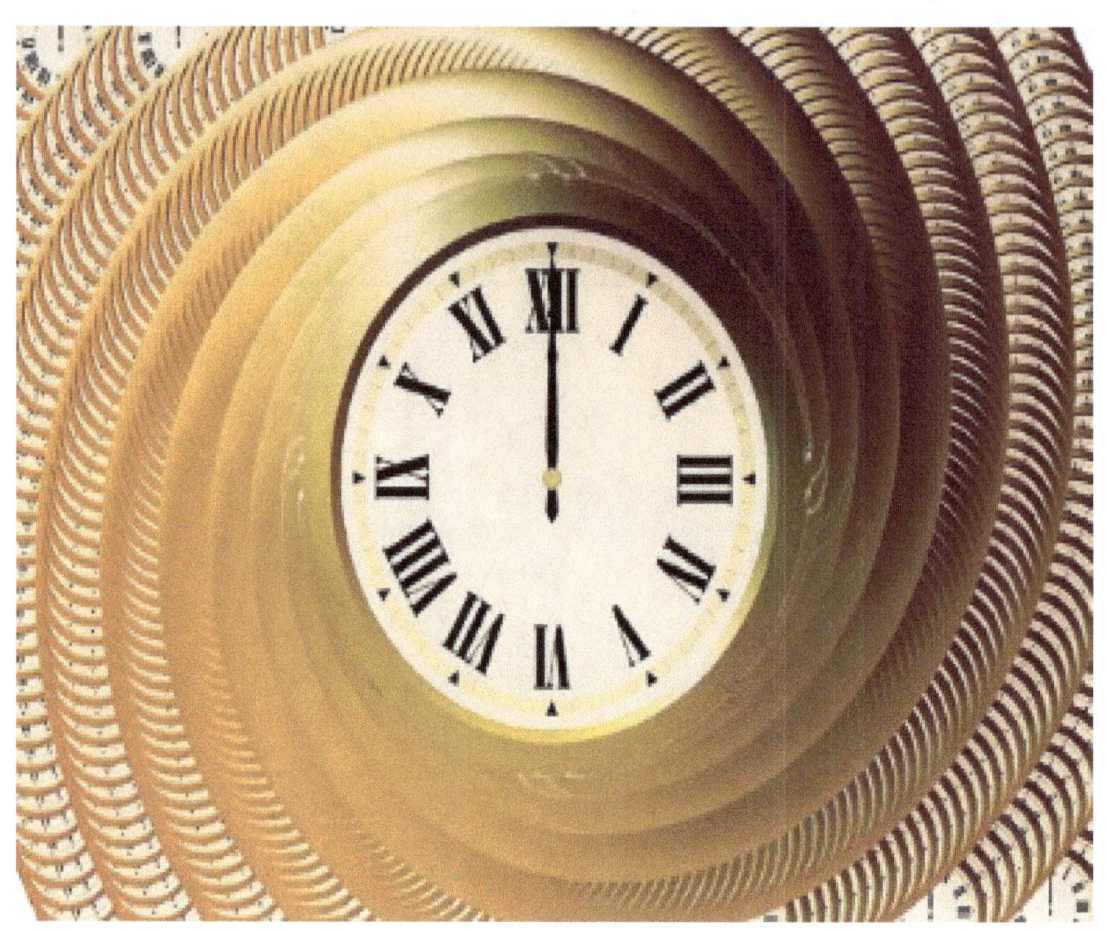

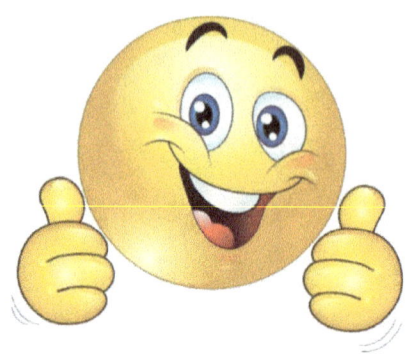

EXCELLENCE in NURSING MATH REVIEW

Mg / Hr

With this formula, the *x factor* and drug concentrations are the same.

Ativan (lorazepam)

A controlled scheduled IV substance, which is used to treat anxiety.

Range: 1 to 20 mg / hr

Premixed solutions: 80 mg / 80 mL   40 mg / 100 mL   20 mg / 250 mL

Ordered: 2 mg / hr

Determine drug concentration: 40 mg / 100 mL = 0.4 mg / mL = (xf)

Determine mL / hr = ___ mg / hr (ordered) = ___ mL / hr
                    ___ (drug concentration)

Reconfirm: rate on pump x (drug concentration) = mg / hr

☐ mL / hr x ☐ mg / mL = ☐ mg / hr
              (xf)

Example #2: Ativan

Drug concentration: 80 mg / 80 mL

Ordered: 12 mg / hr

$$X = \frac{\blacksquare \text{ mg} \times 1}{1 \text{ hr}} \times \frac{\blacksquare \text{ mL}}{\blacksquare \text{ mg}} = \blacksquare \text{ mL / hr}$$

- Determine *x factor* = 80 mg / 80 mL = ▇ *xf*

- Double check = ▇ mL / hr x *1xf* = ▇ mg / hr

Bumex (bumetanide)

A loop diuretic and 1 mg of bumex that is equivalent to 40 mg of lasix.

Range: 0.25 to 2 mg / hr

Premixed solutions:　$\dfrac{10 \text{ mg}}{100 \text{ mL}}$　$\dfrac{12 \text{ mg}}{48 \text{ mL}}$　$\dfrac{25 \text{ mg}}{100 \text{ mL}}$

Ordered: 0.7 mg / hr

- Determine *x factor* = 25 mg / 100 mL = ▇ *xf*

- Determine mL / hr = $\dfrac{\blacksquare \text{ mg / hr (ordered)}}{\blacksquare \text{ xf (x factor)}}$ = ▇ mL / hr

- Double check = rate on pump x (*x factor*) = mg / hr

　　　▇ mL / hr x ▇ *xf (x factor)* = ▇ mg / hr

Example #2: Bumex

Drug concentration: 12 mg / 48 mL

Ordered: 1.5 mg / hr

$$X = \frac{\text{___ mg} \times \text{___ mL}}{1 \text{ hr} \quad \text{___ mg}} = \text{___ mL / hr}$$

- Determine *x factor* = ___ mg / ___ mL = ___ *xf*

- Double check = ___ mL / hr x ___ *xf (x factor)* = ___ mg / hr

Cardene SR (nicardipine)

A calcium channel blocker is used to treat chronic stable angina and hypertension.

Range: 0.5 to 15 mg / hr

Premixed solutions: $\frac{20 \text{ mg}}{200 \text{ mL}}$ $\frac{25 \text{ mg}}{250 \text{ mL}}$ $\frac{40 \text{ mg}}{200 \text{ mL}}$

Ordered: 2.5 mg / hr

- Determine *x factor* = 25 mg / 250 mL = ___ *xf*

- Determine mL / hr = $\frac{\text{___ mg / hr (ordered)}}{\text{___ } xf \text{ (x factor)}}$ = ___ mL / hr

- Double check = rate on pump x *(x factor)* = mg / hr

    ___ mL / hr x ___ *xf (x factor)* = ___ mg / hr

Example #2: Cardene SR

Premixed solution: 40 mg / 200 mL

Ordered: ▮ mg / hr

Infusion pump: 50 mL / hr

- Determine *x factor* = ▮ mg / ▮ mL = ▮ *xf*

- Determine mg / hr = ▮ mL / hr x ▮ *xf (x factor)* = ▮ mg / hr

- Double check = ▮ mg / hr = ▮ mL / hr
                  ▮ *x factor*

EXCELLENCE in NURSING MATH REVIEW

Cardizem (diltiazem hydrochloride)

A calcium channel blocker is used to treat atrial arrhythmia such as fibrillation or flutter.

Range: 5 to 15 mg / hr

Premixed solutions: $\dfrac{100 \text{ mg}}{100 \text{ mL}}$ $\dfrac{125 \text{ mg}}{100 \text{ mL}}$ $\dfrac{250 \text{ mg}}{125 \text{ mL}}$

Ordered: 8 mg / hr

$X = \dfrac{\_\_\_ \text{ mg}}{\text{hr}} \times \dfrac{\_\_\_ \text{ mL}}{250 \text{ mg}} = \_\_\_ \text{ mL / hr}$

- Determine *x factor* = ___ mg / ___ mL = ___ *xf*

- Double check = ___ mL / hr x ___ *xf (x factor)* = ___ mg / hr

Lasix (furosemide)

A loop diuretic which maintains fluid electrolyte balance, improves oxygenation, reduces blood circulation, and decreases high blood pressure.

Range: 20 to 160 mg / hr

Premixed solutions: 100 mg / 100 mL
                               200 mg / 200 mL

Ordered: 40 mg / hr

$$X = \frac{\_\_\_ \text{ mg}}{\text{hr}} \times \frac{\_\_\_ \text{ mL}}{\_\_\_ \text{ mg}} = \_\_\_ \text{ mL / hr}$$

- Determine *x factor* = 100 mg / 100 mL = ___ *xf*

- Double check = ___ mL / hr x ___ *xf (x factor)* = ___ mg / hr

EXCELLENCE in NURSING MATH REVIEW

Narcan (naloxone hydrochloride)

A reversal agent for narcotic overdose with induced respiratory depression patients.

Range: 0.25 to 6.25 mg / hr

Premixed solutions: 4 mg / 250 mL
                             2 mg / 500 mL

Ordered: 0.4 mg / hr

$$X = \frac{0.4 \text{ mg} \times 500 \text{ mL}}{\text{hr} \quad 2 \text{ mg}} = \underline{} \text{ mL / hr}$$

- Determine *x factor* = 2 mg / 500 mL = _____ xf

- Double check = rate on pump x *(x factor)* = mg / hr

    _____ mg / hr x _____ xf *(x factor)* = _____ mg / hr

Protonix (pantoprazole sodium)

This medication is used to treat erosive esophagitis yet not intended for immediate relief of heartburn symptoms.

Range: Check physician's order, pharmacy, and hospital policy.

Remember that these are practice problems.

Premixed solution: 80 mg / 100 mL

Ordered: 8 mg / hr

- Calculate *x factor* = 80 mg / 100 mL = ▒ *xf*

- Determine mL / hr = ▒ mg / hr (ordered) = ▒ mL / hr
  　　　　　　　　　　　▒ *xf (x factor)*

- Double check = rate on pump *x (x factor)* = mg / hr

  ▒ mL / hr x ▒ *xf (x factor)* = ▒ mg / hr

EXCELLENCE in NURSING MATH REVIEW

Theo-24 (theophylline) (aminophylline)

It is used to treat asthma, bronchitis, and COPD (chronic obstructive pulmonary disease).

The signs of toxicity are tremors, nausea, vomiting, and rapid pulse rate.

Range: 4 to 70 mg / hr

Premixed solutions: 500 mg / 500 mL
                                    250 mg / 100 mL

Ordered 13 mg / hr

- Determine *x factor* = 250 mg / 100 mL = ▓ *xf*

- Determine mL / hr = $\dfrac{\text{▓ mg / hr (ordered)}}{\text{▓ }xf\ (x\ factor)}$ = ▓ mL / hr

- Double check = rate on pump x *(x factor)* = mg / hr

    ▓ mL / hr x ▓ *xf (x factor)* = ▓ mg / hr

Note: Theophylline dose equals 80 percent of aminophylline dose.

Answer Sheet

(Mg / hr)

Drugs	X factor	mL / hr	Concentration (mg / mL)
Ativan #1	0.4	5	0.4
#2	1	12	1
Bumetanide #1	0.25	2.8	0.25
#2	*	6	*
Nicardipine	0.1	25	0.1
Cardene #1	0.1	25	0.2
#2	0.2	10 (mg / hr)	0.2
Diltiazem	2	4	2
Furosemide	1	40	1
Naloxone	0.004	100	0.004
Pantoprazole	0.8	10	0.8
Theophylline	2.5	13	2.5

Valium (diazepam)

A short-term benzodiazepine derivative used to treat anxiety disorders, alcohol withdrawal symptoms, or muscle spasms.

Range: 2 to 20 mg / hr

Premixed solution: $\dfrac{100 \text{ mg}}{500 \text{ mL}}$

Ordered: 17 mg / hr

- Determine *x factor*: 100 mg / 500 mL = ▊ *xf*

- Determine mL / hr = $\dfrac{▊ \text{ mg / hr (ordered)}}{▊ \text{ xf (x factor)}}$ = ▊ mL / hr

- Double check = rate on pump x *(x factor)* = mg / hr

    ▊ mL / hr x ▊ *xf (x factor)* = ▊ mg / hr

Versed (midazolam)

This medication is classified as benzodiazepine. It is used to sedate a patient or client who is scheduled for minor surgery, dental work, or other medical procedures. Also used to relieve apprehension.

Premixed solutions: 100 mg / 50 mL
                          50 mg / 100 mL
                          100 mg / 100 mL

Range: 1 to 10 mg / hr

Ordered: 4 mg / hr

- Determine x factor = 100 mg / 50 mL = ▒ xf

- Determine mL / hr = ▒ mg / hr (ordered) = ▒ mL / hr
                                   ▒ xf *(x factor)*

- Double check = rate on pump x *(x factor)* = mg / hr

     ▒ mL / hr x ▒ xf *(x factor)* = ▒ mg / hr

Answer Sheet

(Mg / hr)

Drugs	X factor	mL / hr	Concentration (mg / mL)
Diazepam			
	0.2x		
		85 mL	
			17 mg
Midazolam			
	2x		
		2 mL	
			4 mg

Bonus Problems

1. Angiomax (mg / kg / hr)
2. Dopamine (mcg / kg / min)
3. Fentanyl (mcg / hr)
4. Heparin (units / kg / hr)
5. Insulin (units / kg / hr)
6. Morphine (mg / hr)
7. Oxytocin (mU / min)
8. Precedex (mcg / kg / hr)
9. Solumedrol (mg / kg / hr)
10. Vasopressin (units / min)

practice

practice

practice

practice

Angiomax (bivalirudin)

An anticoagulant used with unstable angina clients who are candidates for surgical percutaneous coronary intervention (PCI) and percutaneous transluminal coronary angioplasty (PCTA).

Range: 0.25 mg to 1.75 mg / kg / hr

Drug concentrations: 250 mg / 50 mL

500 mg / 100 mL

Weight: 120 kg

Ordered: 1.75 mg / kg / hr

Hint: If the dosage calculation is in mg / kg / hr, *remove* 60 minutes (hr) from the formula.

No *x factor* needed

- Determine mL / hr = ☐ mg (ordered) x ☐ kg x 50 mL = ☐ mL/hr
    hr   250 mg
- Double check: 42 mL x 250 mg = ▨ mg / kg / hr
    hr   50 mL   120 kg

Dopamine (no pump but gravity)

Drug concentration: 800 mg / 250 mL = 3200 mcg / mL

Pt's weight: 187 lbs (85 kg)

Microset: 60 gtt

Physician ordered: 10 mcg / kg / min

      gtt / min to gravity

$$X = \frac{10 \text{ mcg (ordered)} \times 85 \text{ kg} \times 60 \text{ min}}{3200 \text{ mcg / mL (drug concentration)}} = \text{gtt / min}$$

Short formula: $\dfrac{\text{dose (mcg} \times \text{kg)} \times 60 \text{ gtt set}}{3200 \text{ mcg / mL}} = 53.3$

Note: As for the short formula, the drip set and concentration are constant, so divide 3200 mcg into 60 gtt set. This may result in certain problems such as dopamine.

X = 10 mcg x 85kg / 53.3 =   gtt / min (or mL / hr)

Dopamine pump rates of titration levels

A vasostimulant administered for the treatment of hypotension, bradycardia, and cardiac arrest.

- Low infusion rates (0.5–2 mcg/kg/min) cause vasodilation, including in the kidneys, which may increase urinary flow.

- Intermediate rates (2 to 10 mcg/kg/min) are associated with stimulation of myocardial contractility, resulting in increased cardiac output.

- **Higher** dosage rates (10 to 20 mcg/kg/min) may result in vasoconstriction and lead to elevated blood pressure.

Fentanyl Citrate (sublimaze)

A narcotic opioid analgesic which works in the brain and nervous system to assist with anesthesia and reduce pain. This is ten times more potent than morphine and shorter duration of action.

Concentrations:
5000 mcg	2500 mcg	1000 mcg	1250 mcg
50 mL	100 mL	100 mL	250 mL

Range: 25 to 200 mcg / hr

Weight: 252 lbs (____ kg)

Ordered: 30 mcg / hr

- Calculate $x\ factor = 1000\ mcg\ /\ 100\ mL = 10\ xf$

- Determine $mL\ /\ hr = \dfrac{30\ mcg\ \times\ 100\ mL}{hr\ \ \ \ \ \ 1000\ mcg} = $ ____ mL / hr

- Double check: rate on pump x ($x\ factor$) = mcg / hr

  ____ mL / hr x ____ xf ($x\ factor$) = ____ mcg / hr

Example #2: Fentanyl

Ordered: 25 mcg / hr

Available: 1 mg / 100 mL NS

Goal: ▓ mL / hr

X = mL / hr: $\dfrac{25 \text{ mcg}}{\text{hr}} \times \dfrac{1 \text{ mg}}{▓ \text{ mcg}} \times \dfrac{▓ \text{ mL}}{1 \text{ mg}} = ▓$ mL / hr

X = mL / hr: $\dfrac{25 \text{ mcg / hr}}{10 \text{ mcg / mL}} = ▓$ mL / hr

✚ Double check: ▓ mL / hr x drug concentration = ▓ mcg / hr

Example #3: Fentanyl

Infusing: 20 mL / hr

On hand: 400 mg / 500 mL (800 mcg / mL)

Goal: ▓ mcg / hr

X = $\dfrac{20 \text{ mL}}{\text{hr}} \times \dfrac{400 \text{ mg}}{▓ \text{ mL}} \times \dfrac{▓ \text{ mcg}}{▓ \text{ mg}} = ▓$ mcg / hr

Heparin

Standard IV

Heparin is an anticoagulant or blood thinner that prevents the formation of blood clots. It is used to treat possible clotting of blood in the veins, arteries, or lungs. This medication is usually initiated before surgery to reduce the risk of blood clots.

- **aPTT**
  - **activated partial thromboplastin time**
  - measures the effectiveness of the 'intrinsic' and common coagulation pathways
    - detects abnormalities in blood clotting
    - monitors the treatment effects of heparin
  - Normal range = 25-39 secs (depends on the lab)

Role of PT, PTT: Warfarin, Heparin Monitoring

Anticoagulant	PT	aPTT
Heparin	Normal	Prolonged
Warfarin (Coumadin)	Prolonged	Normal

Example Only

Warfarin (Coumadin)

- **Indication:** Treatment of venous thrombosis, pulmonary embolis, and thromboembolic disorder
  - Not generally used for DVT/PE prophylaxis (except long term prevention, such as patients with valve replacements) due to delayed onset of action and higher risk of bleeding complications
- **Dose:**
  - Typical starting dose is 2.5 to 5 mg
  - Use "bridge therapy" (LMWH or heparin + warfarin) when immediate anticoagulation is warranted

Example Only

Heparin

Drug concentrations: 10,000 units / 250 mL
12,500 units / 250 mL
25,000 units / 500 mL

Range: 400 to 1,600 units / hr

12 to 18 units / kg / hr (weight based)

Weight: 177 lbs (▨ kg)

Available: 25,000 units / 500 mL

Bolus: 75 units / kg

Ordered: 12 units / kg / hr

1. bolus units = $\dfrac{75 \text{ units}}{\text{kg}} \times \dfrac{\text{▨ kg}}{1} = \text{▨ units}$

2. units / hr = $\dfrac{\text{▨ units}}{\text{▨ kg / hr}} \times \dfrac{\text{▨ kg}}{1} = \text{▨ units / hr}$

3. mL / hr = $\dfrac{\text{▨ units}}{\text{hr}} \times \dfrac{\text{▨ mL}}{25{,}000 \text{ units}} = \text{▨ mL / hr}$

EXCELLENCE in NURSING MATH REVIEW

Heparin Nomogram

1. Baseline investigations: CBC, electrolytes, platelets, INR
2. Give heparin 25,000 units in 500 ml D5W IV start at 1000 units/hr (20 ml/hr)
3. Initial bolus: ☐ None ☐ 2,500 units ☐ 5,000 units

APTT (seconds)	Additional heparin dose	Stop infusion (minutes)	Rate change based on 50 units/mL	Repeat APTT
< 50	☐ 2500 units ☐ 5000 units Bolus over 5–15 minutes	0	+ 3 mL (increase by 150 units/hr)	6 hours
50 - 59	0	0	+ 2 mL (increase by 100 units/hr)	6 hours
60 - 80	0	0	0 (no change)	Next a.m.
81 - 95	0	0	– 1 mL (decrease by 50 units/hr)	6 hours
96 - 110	0	30	– 2 mL (decrease by 100 units/hr)	6 hours
> 110	0	60	– 3 mL (decrease by 150 units/hr)	6 hours

APTT: Activated partial thromboplastin time; CBC: Complete blood count; INR: International normalized ratio

Example Only

The following questions are based on the heparin nomogram.

Ordered: 1,000 units / hr

Available: 25,000 units / 500 mL

$$X = mL/hr = \frac{1000 \text{ units} \times 500 \text{ mL}}{25{,}000 \text{ units}} = \underline{\quad} \text{ mL/hr}$$

- After 6 hrs the PTT is 57, change the rate per nomogram

$$X = \frac{\underline{\quad} \text{ units} \times 500 \text{ mL}}{hr \quad 25{,}000 \text{ units}} = \underline{\quad} \text{ mL/hr}$$

- The 2nd PTT results are > 100 after 6 hrs, change the rate per nomogram.

$$X = \frac{\underline{\quad} \text{ units} \times 500 \text{ mL}}{hr \quad \underline{\quad} \text{ units}} = \underline{\quad} \text{ mL/hr}$$

Example #3: Heparin

Available: 30,000 units / 250 mL

Ordered: 40 mL / hr

How many units / hr via infusion pump?

units / hr = $\dfrac{\text{mL}}{\text{hr}} \times \dfrac{\text{units}}{250 \text{ mL}}$ = units/ hr

Example #4: Heparin

Ordered: 700 units / hr

Available: 12,500 units / 250 mL (50 units / mL)

- Determine mL / hr = $\dfrac{700 \text{ units}}{\text{hr}} \times \dfrac{\text{mL}}{\text{units}}$ = mL / hr

- Check for accuracy = mL / hr x $\dfrac{\text{units}}{\text{mL}}$ = units / hr

Example #5: Heparin

Ordered: Heparin 100 units / hr

Available: 10,000 units / 50 mL (200 units / mL)

Pt's weight: 75 kg (Is this needed in the equation?)

How much mL / hr via infusion pump?

mL / hr = $\dfrac{100 \text{ units}}{\text{hr}} \times \dfrac{50 \text{ mL}}{10,000 \text{ units}}$ = ▮ mL / hr

Example #6: Heparin

Ordered: 18 units / kg / hr

Available: 25,000 units / 500 ml (50 units / mL)

Client's weight : 130 lbs (59 kg)

X = $\dfrac{130 \text{ lb}}{2.2 \text{ lb}} \times \dfrac{1}{\text{kg}} \times \dfrac{18 \text{ units}}{\text{hr}} \times \dfrac{500 \text{ mL}}{25,000 \text{ units}}$ = ▮ mL / hr

X = $\dfrac{18 \text{ units} \times \text{▮ kg / hr}}{50 \text{ units / mL}}$ = ▮ mL / hr

x factor = 25,000 units / 59 kg / ▮ mL = 0.847*xf*

Ordered: $\dfrac{18 \text{ units / kg / hr}}{0.847xf}$ = ▮ mL / hr

Management of Diabetes

- Diet
- Exercise
- Oral Medication
- Insulin Therapy: injection of exogenous insulin analogs when blood glucose levels are high

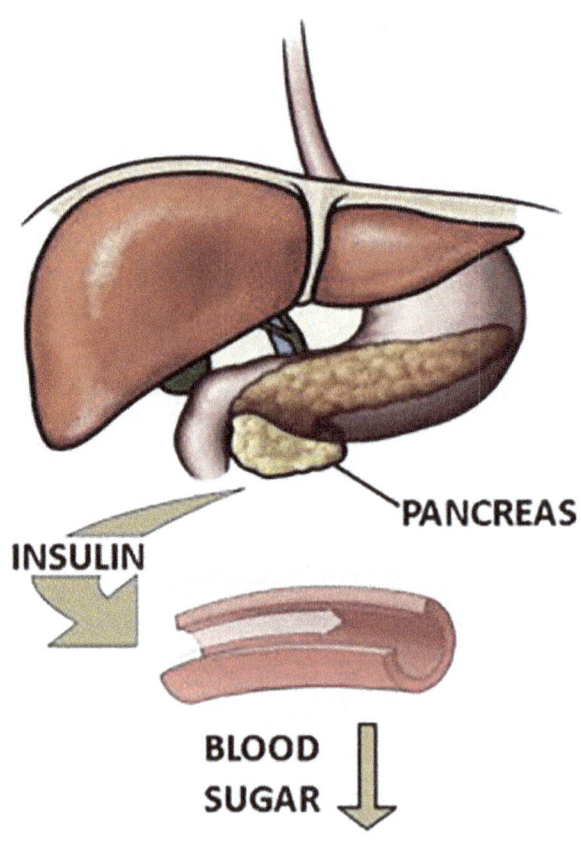

Example Only

EXCELLENCE in NURSING MATH REVIEW

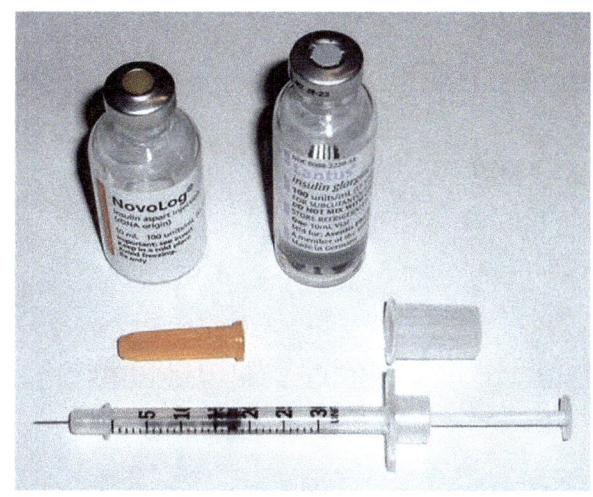

	Type	Trade Name	Onset	Peak	Duration
Rapid Acting	**aspart** **glulisine** **lipsro**	NovoRapid Apidra Humalog	10-15m	1-1.5h	3-5h
Short Acting	**Regular**	Humulin-R Novolin	30-45m	2-3h	6.5h
Intermediate	**NPH**	Humulin-N Novolin	1-3h	5-8h	14-18h
Long Acting	**detemir** **glargine**	Levemir Lantus	1-2h 1-2h	8-10h no peak	12-24h 22-24h

Example Only

Insulin (Regular)

A fast-acting form of hormone insulin, which helps the body to use sugar properly by lowering the amount of glucose in the blood.

Premixed solutions: $\dfrac{100 \text{ units}}{100 \text{ mL}}$ $\dfrac{250 \text{ units}}{250 \text{ mL}}$ $\dfrac{100 \text{ units}}{500 \text{ mL}}$

Range: per physician order and facility policy

Weight: 55 kg

Ordered: 0.2 unit / kg / hr

- Determine units / hr = 0.2 unit x ▩ kg = ▩ units / hr

- Determine the rate to set the IV pump.

    $\dfrac{500 \text{ mL}}{100 \text{ units}}$ x $\dfrac{\text{▩ units}}{\text{hr}}$ = ▩ mL / hr

- Verify accuracy

    $\dfrac{\text{▩ units / hr}}{\text{▩ mL / hr}}$ = ▩ units / kg / hr

EXCELLENCE in NURSING MATH REVIEW

Example #2: Insulin

Ordered: 12 units / hr

Available: 50 units / 100 mL (0.5 unit / mL)

Goal: ____ mL / hr

mL / hr = (12 units × 100 mL) / (hr × ____ units) = ____ mL / hr

Double check: ____ mL / hr × 0.5 unit / mL = ____ units / hr

Practice makes Perfect

Example #3

Insulin GTT Protocol

Formula (BG-60) x 0.03 = number of insulin units / hr

BG = current blood glucose

60 = minutes

Multiplier = 0.03

Target Range for BG:

Low target 70 to 100

High target 110 to 40

Instructions:

    A. If BG is greater than high target, then increase multiplier by 0.01.

    B. If BG is less than low target, then decrease multiplier by 0.01.

    C. If BG is within target range, then no change in multiplier.

    D. BG is recalculated every hour and obtain lab glucose if < 40 or > 600.

Result of Blood Glucose

Initial BG 327 (started on insulin drip protocol) Physician order: target goal 85–110 blood glucose

Mixed solution: 100 units / 100 mL (regular insulin only)

Check every one hour and adjust per protocol.

1. (BG 327–60) x 0.03 = 8 units / hr
2. (BG 277–60) x 0.04 = 9 units / hr
3. (BG 167–60) x 0.05 = 5 units / hr
4. (BG 110–60) x 0.05 = 3 units / hr (no change)
5. Target goal range was met then contact physician for additional orders.

Let's Practice

1. BG of 327 with 8 units / hr

   Determine rate to set infusion pump per mL / hr

   $$X = \frac{\_\_\_ \text{ units}}{\text{hr}} \times \frac{\_\_\_ \text{ mL}}{\_\_\_ \text{ units}} = \_\_\_ \text{ mL / hr}$$

2. BG of 110 with 3 units / hr

   Mixed solution: 50 units / 100 mL

   Determine rate = ___ mL / hr

   $$X = \frac{\_\_\_ \text{ units}}{\text{hr}} \times \frac{\_\_\_ \text{ mL}}{\_\_\_ \text{ units}} = \_\_\_ \text{ mL / hr}$$

practice

practice

practice

practice

Morphine Sulphate

Morphine is considered a controlled schedule II substance that is used to treat severe pain, which reduces respiratory respirations.

Range: 1 to 10 mg / hr

Premixed solutions: 250 mg / 50 mL
                            100 mg / 100 mL

Ordered: 2 mg / hr

    A) Calculate x factor = 250 mg / 50 mL = ☐ xf

    B) Determine mL / hr = $\dfrac{\text{▇ mg / hr (ordered)}}{\text{▇ } xf \text{ (}x \text{ factor)}}$ = ▇ mL / hr

    C) Check for accuracy = rate on pump x (x factor) = mg / hr

        ▇ mL / hr x ▇ xf (x factor) = ▇ mg / hr

    mL / hr = $\dfrac{\text{▇ mg } \times \text{ ▇ mL}}{\text{hr } \quad \text{▇ mg}}$ = ▇ mL / hr

Pitocin (oxytocin)

This medication is indicated for medical verses an elective induction of labor. Oxytocin helps to improve uterine contraction, control post- partum bleeding or hemorrhage. Be sure to monitor the fetal heart rate.

Range: 0.5 to 10 mU / mL

Available: 30 units / 500 mL
            40 units / 1000 mL

Ordered: 8 milliunits / min

Determine: ___ mL / hr via infusion pump.

$$X = \frac{8 \text{ mU}}{\text{min}} \times \frac{60 \text{ min}}{1 \text{ hr}} \times \frac{1 \text{ unit}}{1000 \text{ mU}} \times \frac{500 \text{ mL}}{30 \text{ units}} = \underline{\quad} \text{ mL / hr}$$

Infusing: 2.3 mL / hr

Available: 40 units / 1000 mL

Determine: ___ mU / min via pump

$$\text{mU / min} = \frac{\underline{\quad} \text{ mL}}{\text{hr}} \times \frac{1 \text{ hr}}{\underline{\quad} \text{ min}} \times \frac{\underline{\quad} \text{ units}}{\underline{\quad} \text{ mL}} \times \frac{\underline{\quad} \text{ mU}}{1 \text{ unit}} = \underline{\quad} \text{ mU / min}$$

Precedex (dexmedetomdine)

Classified as a selective sedative in the alpha 2-adrenegic agonist. This medication indicates sedated or initially intubated and mechanically ventilated patients. Not to be used greater than 24 hours.

Range: 0.2 to 1.5 mcg / kg / hr

Drug concentrations: 200 mcg / 50 mL (**4 mcg / mL**)
                            400 mcg / 100 mL

Pt's weight: 165 lbs (▓ kg)

Ordered: 0.7 mcg / kg / hr

$$X = \frac{0.7 \text{ mcg}}{\text{kg / hr}} \times \frac{\blacksquare \text{ kg}}{1} \times \frac{\blacksquare \text{ mL}}{\blacksquare \text{ mcg}} = \blacksquare \text{ mL/ hr}$$

- Calculate *x factor* = $\frac{4 \text{ mcg} / 75 \text{ kg}}{\text{mL}}$ = ▓ *xf*

- Determine mL / hr = $\frac{0.7 \text{ mcg / kg / hr}}{\blacksquare \text{ } x \text{ factor}}$ = ▓ mL / hr

- Double check for accuracy = rate on pump x (*x factor*) = mcg / kg / hr

    ▓ mL / hr x ▓ *xf* (*x factor*) = ▓ mcg / kg / hr

Solumedrol (methylprednisolone sodium succinate)

A corticosteroid, hormone, and potent anti-inflammatory medication that is used for life-threatening or septic shock and acute spinal cord injury. The goal is to improve or sustain neurological status.

Drug concentrations: 50 mg / 100 mL (0.5 mg / mL)
$\qquad$ 100 mg / 100 mL
$\qquad$ 500 mg / 250 mL

Weight: 70 kg

Ordered: 0.05 mg / kg / hr

$$X = \frac{[] \text{ ordered} \times [] \text{ kg} \times [] \text{ mL}}{\text{hr} \quad\quad\quad 50 \text{ mg}} = [] \text{ mL/ hr}$$

Example #2: Solumedrol

Ordered: 1.6 mg / kg / hr

Weight: 55 kg

Solution: 500 mg / 250 mL

$$X = \frac{[] \text{ mg} \times [] \text{ kg / hr}}{[] \text{ concentration}} = [] \text{ mL / hr}$$

Example #3: Solumedrol

Determine: ▓ mg / kg / hr

IV infusing @ 44 mL / hr

Solution: 500 mg / 250 mL

Weight: 55 kg

mg / kg / hr = ▓ mL x ▓ mg x 1 = ▓ mg / kg / hr
　　　　　　　　hr　 ▓ mL　 ▓ kg

Example #4: Solumedrol

Determine: ▓ mL / hr

Solution: 100 mg / 100 mL

Weight: 220 lbs

Ordered: 0.1 mg / kg / hr

X = 0.1 mg x 100 kg / hr = ▓ mL / hr
　　　▓ concentration

Pitressin (vasopressin)

A vasopressor used in the treatment of acute lower GI hemorrhage, vasodilated shock, and variceal bleed. No longer used in the ACLS protocol. Also classified as an ADH pituitary hormone.

DO NOT
DO NOT
DO NOT TITRATE
DO NOT

Pitressin

Premixed solutions: 50 units / 50 mL
20 units / 100 mL
250 units / 250 mL
200 units / 500 mL

Range: 0.01 to 0.09 units / min

Ordered: 0.04 units / min

Determine: ___ mL / hr

$$X = \frac{\text{___ units (ordered)}}{\text{min}} \times \frac{60 \text{ min}}{1 \text{ hr}} \times \frac{\text{___ x 100 mL}}{\text{___ units}} = \text{___ mL / hr}$$

Bonus Answer Sheet

1. **Bivalirudin (mg / kg / hr)**
   x factor = 0.041*xf*
   42 mL / hr
   drug concentration = 5 mg / mL

2. **Dopamine (mcg / kg / min)**
   x factor = .627*xf*
   16 gtt / min
   drug concentration = 53.3 mcg / mL

3. **Sublimaze # 1 (mcg / hr)**
   x factor = 10*xf*
   3 mL / hr
   drug concentration = 10 mcg / mL

   ➢ 2.5 mL / hr
      drug concentration = 10 mcg / mL

   ➢ 16,000 mcg / hr

4. **Heparin (unit / kg / hr)**
   bolus = 6300 units
   964.8 units / hr
   mL / hr = 19.3

5. **Heparin Nanogram (unit / hr)**
   20 mL / hr
   22 mL / hr and 1100 units
   Stop infusion for 30 minutes, 20 mL and 1000 units

EXCELLENCE in NURSING MATH REVIEW

6. **Heparin**
   - 4800 units / hr
   - 14 mL / hr
   - 0.5 mL / hr
     - ❖ 21.3 mL / hr
     - ❖ 21.2 mL / hr (depends on calculator)
     - ❖ *0.847xf*
     - ❖ 23.3 mL / hr

7. **Human Insulin (unit / kg / hr)**
   11 units / hr

   55 mL / hr

   0.2 units / kg / hr

8. **Regular Insulin**
   24 mL / hr

   12 units / hr

9. **Insulin Protocol**
   8 mL / hr

   6 mL / hr

10. **Morphine (mg / hr)**

5 *x factor*

0.4 mL / hr

5 mg / mL (drug concentration)

11. **Oxytocin (mU / min)**
    - 8 mL / hr
    - 60 mU / mL (drug concentration)
    - 1.5 mU / min

12. **Dexmedetomdine (mcg / kg / hr)**
    13.1 mL / hr

    0.053*xf*

    13.1 mL / hr

    mcg / kg / hr = 0.7

13. **Methylprednisolone (mg / kg / hr)**
    7 mL / hr

    44 mL / hr

    1.6 mg / kg / hr

    10 mL / hr

14. **Vasopressin (units / min) = 12 mL / hr**

Interpretation of Acid Base Gases
Arterial Blood Gases (ABGs)

R Respiratory   pH ↑ PCO2 ↓ Alkalosis

O Opposite   pH ↓ PCO2 ↑ Acidosis

M Metabolic   pH ↑ HCO3 ↑ Alkalosis

E Equal   pH ↓ HCO3 ↓ Acidosis

Uncompensated: CO2 or HCO3 normal
Partially Compensated: Nothing is normal
Compensated: pH is normal (7.4 baseline/neutral)

Compromised individuals:

1. pH and HCO_3^- are "happy friends" they like to go in the same direction.

2. CO_2 is the "unhappy friends," which pH sprints in the opposite direction when they see each other approaching.

Therefore:

3. Decreased pH with increased CO_2-: Respiratory ACIDOSIS

4. Increased pH with decreased CO_2-: Respiratory ALKALOSIS

5. Decreased pH with decreased HCO_3^-: Metabolic ACIDOSIS

6. Increased pH with increased HCO_3^-: Metabolic ALKALOSIS

TANGA C. ELAM, BSN, RN, MSA, BAA

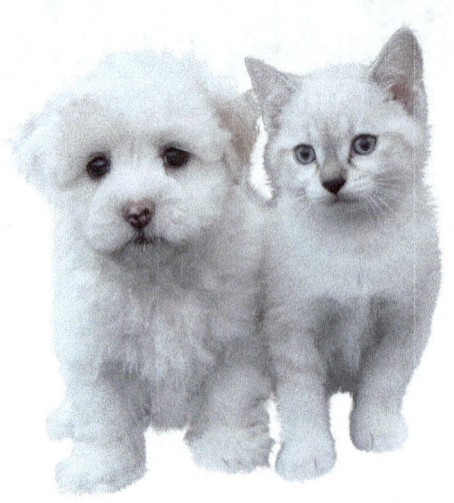

Acidic — Neutral — Basic

7.35 - 7.45
pH

45-35
paCO$_2$
(Respiratory)

22-26
HCO$_3$
(Metabolic)

R Respiratory	PH ↑	PCO$_2$ ↓	Alkalosis
O Opposite	PH ↓	PCO$_2$ ↑	Acidosis
M Metabolic	PH ↑	HCO$_3$ ↑	Alkalosis
E Equal	PH ↓	HCO$_3$ ↓	Acidosis

Compensated: PH is normal (7.4 neutral)
Partially Compensated: ALL abnormal
Uncompensated: Co2 OR HCo3 is Normal

EXCELLENCE in NURSING MATH REVIEW

ABGs Practice Problems:

1. pH: 7.44, $PaCO_2$: 29, HCO_3: 14 _____

2. pH: 7.38, $PaCO_2$: 45, HCO_3: 32 _____

3. pH: 7.45, $PaCO_2$: 45, HCO_3: 22 _____

4. pH: 7.55, $PaCO_2$: 23, HCO_3: 16 _____

5. pH: 7.16, $PaCO_2$: 50, HCO_3: 33 _____

6. pH: 7.75, $PaCO_2$: 34, HCO_3: 32 _____

7. pH: 7.30, $PaCO_2$: 36, HCO_3: 16 _____

8. pH: 7.43, $PaCO_2$: 39, HCO_3: 24 _____

9. pH: 7.53, $PaCO_2$: 49, HCO_3: 30 _____

10. pH: 7.11, $Pa CO_2$: 28, HCO_3: 21 _____

11. pH:7.53, $PaCO_2$: 32, HCO_3: 24 _____

12. pH: 7.56, $PaCO_2$: 24, HCO_3: 23 _____

13. pH: 7.25, $PaCO_2$: 40, HCO_3: 20 _____

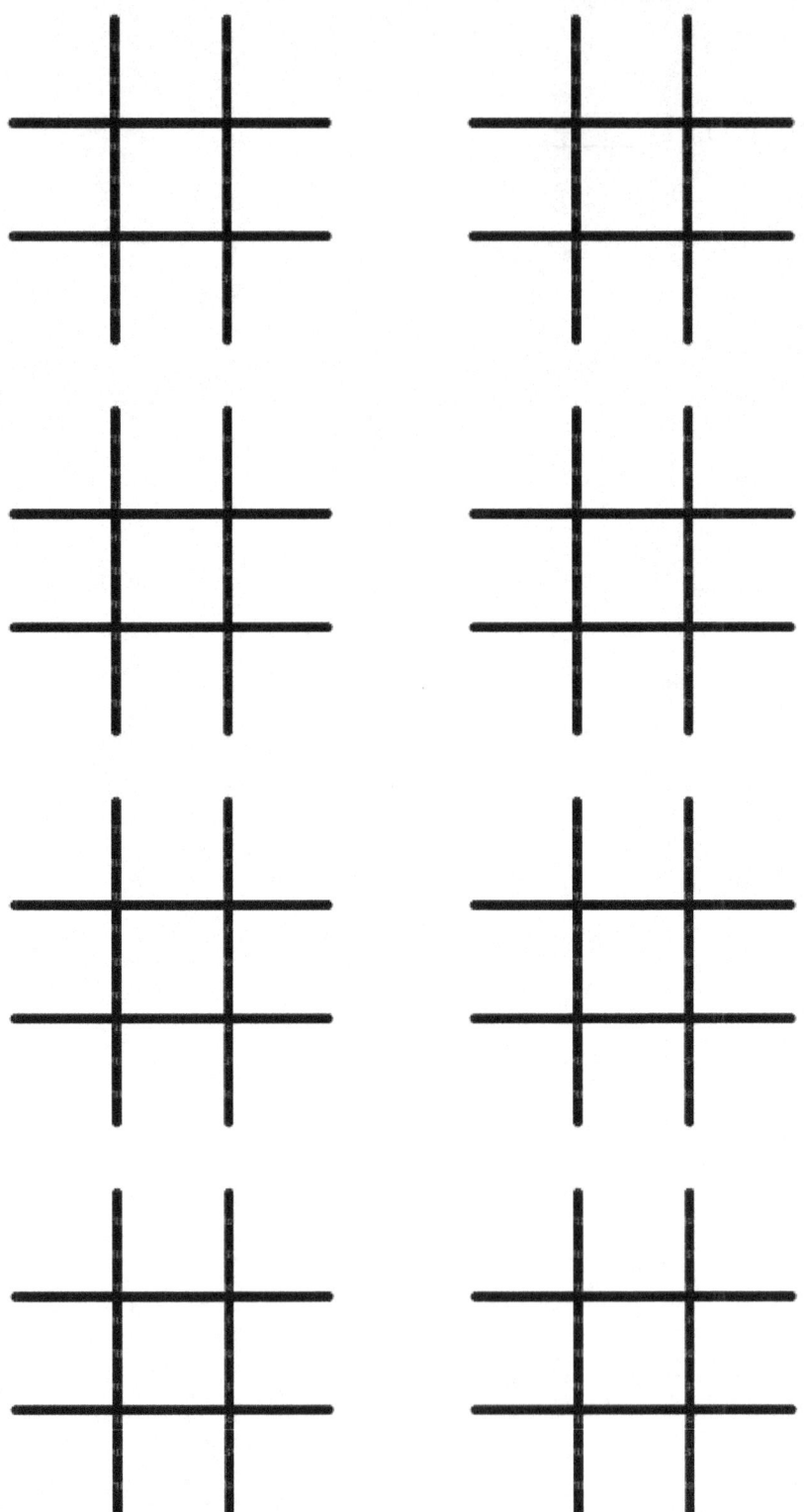

EXCELLENCE in NURSING MATH REVIEW

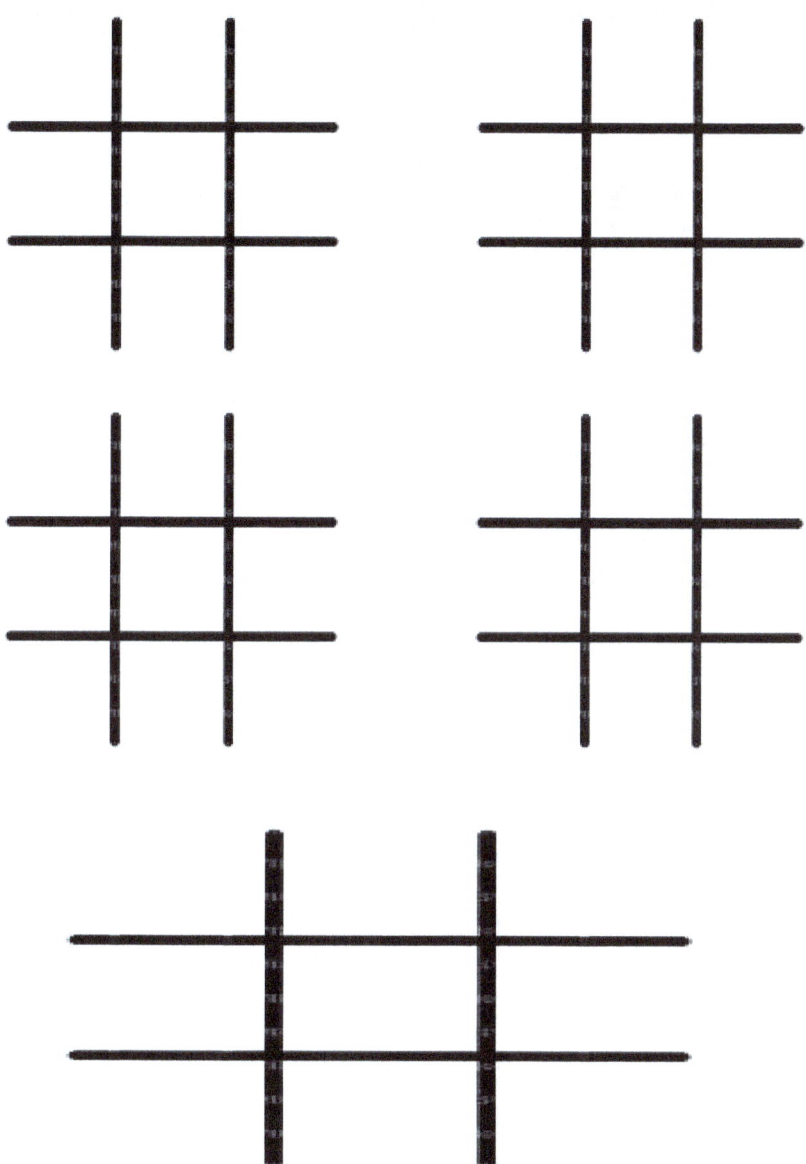

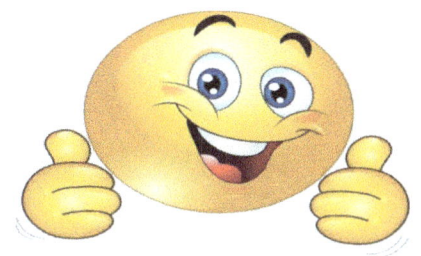

Some Common Causes:

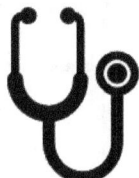

Respiratory Acidosis > respiratory depression, COPD, and pneumonia

Respiratory Alkalosis > hyperventilation, fever, and aspirin poisoning

Metabolic Acidosis > diabetes, shock, and renal failure

Metabolic Alkalosis > $NaHCO_3$ overdose, prolonged emesis, and nasal gastric drainage

Answer Sheet
ABG Interpretations

1. respiratory alkalosis fully compensated

2. respiratory acidosis fully compensated

3. normal

4. respiratory alkalosis partially compensated

5. respiratory acidosis partially compensated

6. metabolic alkalosis uncompensated

7. metabolic acidosis uncompensated

8. normal

9. metabolic alkalosis partially compensated

10. metabolic acidosis partially compensated

11. respiratory alkalosis uncompensated

12. respiratory alkalosis

13. metabolic acidosis

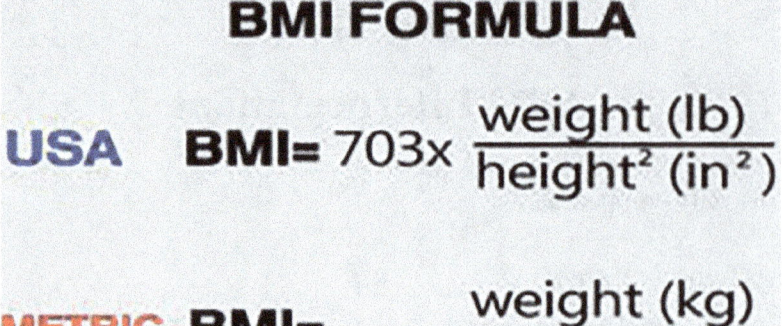

Practice calculating your BMI (body mass index)

Example:

Weight = 170 lbs
Height = 67 inches

BMI Formula: $\dfrac{703 \times 150\,\#}{67 \times 67} = \dfrac{119510}{4489} =$

Weight	lbs	100	105	110	115	120	125	130	135	140	145	150	155	160	165	170	175	180	185	190	195	200	205	210	215
	Kgs	45.5	47.7	50.0	52.3	54.5	56.8	59.1	61.4	63.6	65.9	68.2	70.5	72.7	75.0	77.3	79.5	81.8	84.1	86.4	88.6	90.9	93.2	95.5	97.7
Height in/cm																									
5'00" - 152.4		19	20	21	22	23	24	25	26	27	28	29	30	31	32	33	34	35	36	37	38	39	40	41	42
5'01" - 154.9		18	19	20	21	22	23	24	25	26	27	28	29	30	31	32	33	34	35	36	36	37	38	39	40
5'02" - 157.4		18	19	20	21	22	22	23	24	25	26	27	28	29	30	31	32	33	33	34	35	36	37	38	39
5'03" - 160.0		17	18	19	20	21	22	23	24	24	25	26	27	28	29	30	31	32	32	33	34	35	36	37	38
5'04" - 162.5		17	18	18	19	20	21	22	23	24	24	25	26	27	28	29	30	31	31	32	33	34	35	36	37
5'05" - 165.1		16	17	18	19	20	20	21	22	23	24	25	25	26	27	28	29	30	30	31	32	33	34	35	35
5'06" - 167.6		16	17	17	18	19	20	21	21	22	23	24	25	25	26	27	28	29	29	30	31	32	33	34	34
5'07" - 170.1		15	16	17	18	18	19	20	21	22	22	23	24	25	25	26	27	28	29	29	30	31	32	33	33
5'08" - 172.7		15	16	16	17	18	19	19	20	21	22	22	23	24	25	25	26	27	28	28	29	30	31	32	32
5'09" - 175.2		14	15	16	17	17	18	19	20	20	21	22	22	23	24	25	25	26	27	28	28	29	30	31	31
5'10" - 177.8		14	15	15	16	17	18	18	19	20	20	21	22	22	23	24	25	25	26	27	28	28	29	30	30
5'11" - 180.3		14	14	15	16	16	17	18	18	19	20	21	31	22	23	23	24	25	25	26	27	27	28	29	30
6'00" - 182.8		13	14	14	15	16	17	17	18	19	19	20	21	21	22	23	23	24	25	25	26	27	27	28	29
6'01" - 185.4		13	13	14	15	15	16	17	17	18	19	19	20	21	21	22	23	23	24	25	25	26	27	27	28
6'02" - 187.9		12	13	14	14	15	16	16	17	18	18	19	19	20	21	21	22	23	23	24	25	25	26	27	27
6'03" - 190.5		12	13	13	14	15	15	16	16	17	18	18	19	20	20	21	21	22	23	23	24	25	25	26	26
6'04" - 193.0		12	12	13	14	14	15	15	16	17	17	18	18	19	20	20	21	22	22	23	23	24	25	25	26

Answer: BMI (body mass index) = 26.2 (overweight)

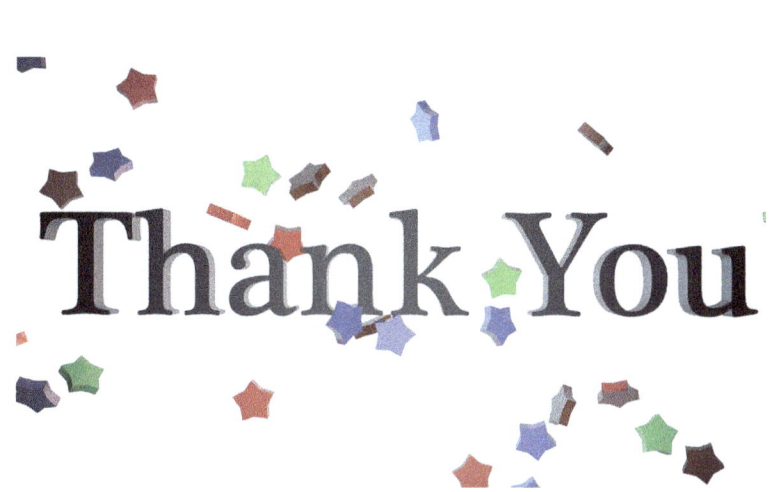

References

Central Carolina Technical College. (n.d.). CCTC – How much can you accomplish? See for yourself. http://www.cctech.edu/

DrofRx. (n.d.). DrofRx.com. http://drofrx.com/

Sonne, J., Goyal, A., & Lopez-Ojeda, W. (2023, July 3). Dopamine. In StatPearls. StatPearls Publishing. https://www.ncbi.nlm.nih.gov/books/NBK535451/

eDucate™ Innovate Research & Development™. (n.d.). [Resource].

RnCeus Interactive. (n.d.). Hemodynamic measurement terminology. http://www.rnceus.com/hemo/term.htm

Hughes, R. G. (2008). Medication administration safety. In R. G. Hughes (Ed.), Patient safety and quality: An evidence-based handbook for nurses. Agency for Healthcare Research and Quality (US). https://www.ncbi.nlm.nih.gov/books/NBK2656/

RX-Success. (n.d.). Intermediate IV practice problems. http://www.austincc.edu/rxsucces/pdf/moduleinterIV_answers.pdf

Lakeman, R. (n.d.). Software and solutions for teaching and learning drug calculations, on-line testing, tutorials, calculators and tests. Alcohol Use Disorders Identification Test (AUDIT) – Sample test. http://testandcalc.com/Drug_Calcs_Desc.html

Karch, A. M. (2011). Lippincott's nursing drug guide. Lippincott Williams & Wilkins.

Luscombe, M. D., Owens, B. D., & Burke, D. (2011). Weight estimation in paediatrics: A comparison of the APLS formula and the formula "Weight = 3(age) + 7." Emergency Medicine Journal, 28(7), 590–593. https://pubmed.ncbi.nlm.nih.gov/20659877/

Allen, M. (2013, September 20). How many die from medical mistakes in U.S. hospitals? NPR. https://www.npr.org/sections/health-shots/2013/09/20/224507654/how-many-die-from-medical-mistakes-in-u-s-hospitals

Review of dosage calculation methods. (n.d.).
http://wps.prenhall.com/wps/media/objects/1145/1173501/dosagecalculations.pdf

SwccITdept. (2011, May 3). Body surface area tutorial [Video]. YouTube.
https://www.youtube.com/watch?v=gHMhgp1xfjc

UMA Pharm Tech. (2014, November 13). *Pediatric dosages and dosing by weight* [Video]. YouTube.
https://www.youtube.com/watch?v=CbXziphqhpk

HealthHearty. (n.d.). *Vascular resistance*

About the Author

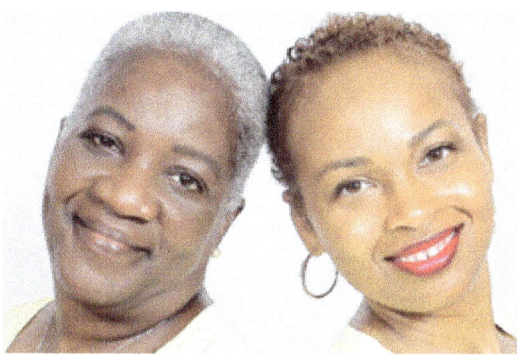

Tanga C. Elam is a certified Woman Minority Veteran CEO of RN Math Excellence, LLC. She is also certified as a Mental Health First-Aider USA. She is highly skilled as an intensive care travel nurse, licensed in seven states for the past twenty-five years. Ms. Elam has taught as an adjunct instructor in the Allied Health Science nursing program for five years.

She holds a master's degree in health service administration and a bachelor's in public health education with a minor in management from Central Michigan University. She also received a second Bachelor of Science degree in nursing from Clayton State University. To complete her education, she also earned an associate degree in science and a licensed practical nursing certificate from Mott Community College.

She has an unpublished thesis titled, "Aspirin Therapy Can Improve Hypertension in Women with Cardiovascular Disease." Ms. Elam wrote her first book Intravenous Math Workbook to Reduce Medication Errors which included application-based practice examples utilizing the *x-factor* guidelines.

The second RNurse Math Workbook is exceptional in achieving a nursing license by reviewing dimensional analysis review before taking the Next Generation NCLEX® examination.

Ms. Elam was awarded a third-place certificate for excellence in communicating a well-developed business plan from Florida's Veterans Entrepreneurship nine-week program. Also, currently an active member of Central Michigan University Black Alumni Chapter, Florida and American Nurses Associations, Talen Charles Brit Scholarship Walk a Thon, Morehouse College Annual Math Competition Bootcamp with Florida Math Mentor Team, American Breast Cancer 5K walk of Florida Blue and Abyssinia Missionary Baptist Church. Reading spiritual books and relaxing near a beautiful koi pond makes her life amazing and more.

TANGA C. ELAM, BSN, RN, MSA, BAA